T5-DHQ-648

PURSUIT OF AGREEMENT
Psychiatry & the Law

PURSUIT OF AGREEMENT
Psychiatry & the Law

By

JONAS B. ROBITSCHER, JD, MD

DISTRICT OF COLUMBIA BAR, UNIVERSITY OF PENNSYLVANIA SCHOOL
OF MEDICINE, THE INSTITUTE OF THE PENNSYLVANIA HOSPITAL,
THE LANKENAU HOSPITAL, PHILADELPHIA, VILLANOVA
UNIVERSITY SCHOOL OF LAW, PENNSYLVANIA

J. B. LIPPINCOTT COMPANY

Philadelphia & Toronto

TO JEAN

Foreword

IF THE LAW is sometimes complex and if psychiatry is sometimes obscure, the area where these disciplines meet and overlap may, understandably, be less than completely clear. This book has grown from the attempt to throw light on the murky area which we call Forensic Psychiatry.

The subject is more understandable if the approach is not—as it often appears to be—piecemeal and if—although they seldom are— legal principles of general application are emphasized. The unifying themes running through the various topics in this book are stressed in the hope that what appear to be illogicalities and inconsistencies will seem more nearly reconcilable and more easily understood. The legal themes that I have stressed are those I feel are the most important historically and most useful for current understanding, although principles I have not stressed may be equally worth emphasizing.

In 1961, the American Bar Foundation published its monumental survey of many crucial areas of Forensic Psychiatry, *The Mentally Disabled and the Law*. This book, the result of five years of work by a large staff, is of surpassing importance in Forensic Psychiatry. This superb source is too extensive for those not intimately involved in the fields it covers, but I have relied heavily on it in the present book. I am deeply indebted to the authors of this Report and to its editors, Frank T. Lindman and Donald M. McIntyre, Jr. While all other authors or editors in the Index of Names are given a page reference for each mention of their work, no attempt has been made to treat Lindman and McIntyre with equal fairness, since the references to their work—cited merely as *Report*—are so multiple.

I would like to express special appreciation to Dr. J. Martin Myers, Medical Director, Institute of the Pennsylvania Hospital, for many of the ideas on commitment and admissions procedures, derived from his lectures to the medical students. I am also indebted to Thomas M. Kerr, Esq., Albert L. Stark, Esq., and to June Miller, Librarian of

7

the Institute of the Pennsylvania Hospital, for critical and research help; to Charles J. Cooper, Esq., Carter Harrison, of J. B. Lippincott Company, and my wife, for editorial services; and to Eleanor Langdon, who typed and read this manuscript.

JONAS B. ROBITSCHER
1 March, 1966

Contents

Law and Psychiatry

L AW is all logic and reason, or at least it sets out to be so. But for a legal system to function, it must be more than merely logical and reasonable. It must be definite. It must be based on precedent. It must rely on rules. And so in the course of time all functioning legal systems become legalistic, and in the process some of the logic and reason gets left behind.

A case concerning a contract comes to court and it is decided "on the merits" of the case and also on the basis of decisions in past cases and—on such a factor as whether so much time has elapsed that the plaintiff, although otherwise having a cause of action, no longer has a cause of action.

Or consider the Louisiana case of a couple that was separated for five months, the wife in Louisiana and the husband in California. They were reconciled, and seven months later a child was born who, according to medical testimony presented in court, was not a seven months' but a fully mature nine months' baby. Since the baby was not conceived at the end of the separation, it must have been conceived before the separation—this was the wife's claim—and thus it represented the outcome of a period of gestation of one year and five days. The court stated that although this is "believed to be a medical impossibility," the child is still legitimate and the father is responsible for his welfare, but on the ground of prematurity instead of postmaturity. A state statute, which holds any child legitimate if husband and wife have been together during a period running from 180 to 300 days before the birth of a child, takes precedence over the best medical testimony. Said the court: "Remoteness is not a ground for disavowal . . . unless the husband and wife have been remote from one another during the entire period of 180–300 days prior to birth."[1]

The court has not been fooled, nor, from a legal point of view, is it being illogical or unreasonable. The policy of the state is to assume legitimacy in order to protect infants, and to this end a statute has been passed. In the interest of the general good, this case must be governed by the statute, even though the judge may have his own private view of the application of the statute to the case before the court.

To the doctor, legitimacy is based on genetic fact; to the lawyer, it is based on legal definition.

And so even though courts pride themselves on logic and reason, if an action has not been filed by the time specified, or if an allegation is not made in the correct language, or if the forms that the law requires have not been adhered to, or if precedent or the words of a statute are controlling, then the logic and the reason do not have a chance to be brought into play.

Psychiatry—and when we use this word in this book, we usually mean modern psychiatry as Freud has left it—deals with the illogical and the unreasonable. Freud's central idea was that human actions have their sources both in the conscious, which may be governed by reason, and the unconscious, which is not governed by reason, by the intellect and logic, and which in fact is by definition *unreasonable*. In attempting to describe and deal with the illogical and unreasonable actions of humans, psychiatrists are somewhat contemptuous of precedent, and they often fail to please the court when asked to categorize and place information in neat cubbyholes in the fashion that lawyers approve.

When these two disciplines meet, therefore, we may expect to find confusion, complexity, and mutual dissatisfaction.

The long, uneasy flirtation between law and medicine is unlikely ever to end in harmonious matrimony with understanding and acceptance of the points of view of each side. At the very best one might foresee some *mariage de convenance* but, more likely, there will be a shotgun wedding forced on the parties concerned by a public impatient both with legal argument and psychiatric differences in open court. Certainly, at times, it has seemed that, rather than there being a happy ending to the courtship, mutual antipathy might lead to an open and irreconcilable breach. Conflicting opinions have been expressed in forthright terms to such a degree that one wonders how far it will ever be possible to bring together in a spirit of mutual toleration two forces, each bent on asserting its own views to the exclusion of the others.[2]

The relationship between law and psychiatry presents difficult and unsolved problems. Perhaps, by their very nature, some of these problems will continue to remain unsolved. Such questions as whether a crime committed under compulsion, that is a crime committed by someone driven by a so-called irresistible impulse, should therefore be declared not a crime raise profound philosophical, moral, and ethical questions, and they also raise psychiatric questions to which we now have no clear answers. Are some impulses irresistible? Is there such a thing as free will? To what extent can or should a court give cognizance to unconscious motives?

In other areas, the relationship between law and psychiatry is less complicated and deals with more practical matters, such as the civil rights of committed patients or the legal ability of such people as the retarded, senile, or psychotic to enter into valid contracts, dispose of real estate, marry, or write valid wills.

Early in the century, when psychiatry was receiving an impetus from the new science of psychoanalysis, there was much hope, some of which has survived, that psychiatrists using psychoanalytic theory could do much to reform the judicial process, rehabilitate criminals, and generally bring about a great enlightenment in certain areas of law, particularly criminal law. During recent years, there has been a reaction to these hopes, and lawyers and judges have been critical of psychiatry because of its failure to be as useful in the judicial process as they had once thought it could be.

Looking at the two, at law and psychiatry, it is not hard to find still other reasons to explain why they do not accommodate more harmoniously. Law tends to be absolutist, psychiatry relativist; law tends to see the world in terms of black and white, psychiatry in gradations. When a robber is brought before the court, although there are degrees of severity of the charges that may be brought or of the sentence set, the basic question is the absolute question of guilt or innocence. Even though it may be reasonably apparent that the accused is guilty, he will have to be set free unless certain legal criteria concerning witnesses and evidence are met.

The psychiatrist sees everything in relative terms. If a patient announces that he has murdered his wife, or has decided to become a medical missionary to a colony of lepers, the psychiatrist will not classify these actions as, respectively, "bad" or "good": he will try to understand and to probe, and in the process he will try not be judgmental. Courts are, of course, judgmental.

Again, law has been developed to protect not only the individual from society but also society from the individual. The psychiatrist is not primarily interested in the individual's relationships to the outside world; he is more concerned with the individual's relationship to various components of his own personality. A psychiatrist can work happily with a thief, a pervert, an addict and—except in those very rare instances where the safety of others seems imminently and crucially threatened—he will feel no responsibility for warning others that a danger is in their midst.

Further, law is a public process, of public record, and this feature allows the great safeguard of judicial review—the review by a superior court of the decision of a lower court—to come into play. A psychiatric relationship, doctor and patient, is based on the old medical tradition of privacy and confidentiality that dates back to Hippocrates and earlier. The essence of a psychiatric relationship is trust in the doctor by the patient, and certainty that statements made will be held confidential is basic to that trust. In modern society, we have seen the emergence of a new species of physician not known in the previous 2,500 years, the court-appointed psychiatrist who examines the prisoner as if he were the prisoner's doctor, asking him for full trust and confidence, then goes to the court—which pays him—and tells what he has learned. Whether a doctor who tries to serve two masters can fulfill his functions to either is a question being asked increasingly.

Dr. Sanford Lewis, a physician who lectures on medicine and law at Rutgers University School of Law, has described the varying functions of medical scientist—psychiatrist and others—and the courts of law:

It is the function of medical scientists to search for truth. It is the obligation of courts of law to delineate justice. These aims are not identical. Eminent psychiatrists may differ as to whether a defendant is mentally competent to stand trial. The bench must make a definitive judgment. Physicians may argue as to whether or not a single trauma can contribute to the development of breast cancer. The court, on the other hand, faced with the cries of an allegedly aggrieved plaintiff, must reach a decision. Scientists may debate, philosophize, and qualify. The law, on the other hand, is burdened with the awesome responsibility of reaching a verdict.[3]

Whitlock has tried to pinpoint some of the factors involved in the conflict between law and psychiatry.

In attempting to bring mutual understanding to the parties concerned in the management of the mentally ill offender it is necessary to examine fundamentals, not the least of which is the language which each side uses in its everyday practice. Both psychiatry and law use a technical language which often makes for confusion over words used in a special manner differing from their normal meaning as defined in ordinary speech. Behind the use of language is a basic philosophy of ideas relating to the human personality and its place in society and the cosmos. . . . Perhaps most fundamental of all is the differing personality structure separating those who become lawyers and those who become doctors. Much could be written on this theme but it is likely that the known facts barely justify the speculations.

Undoubtedly the psychiatrist is so directly concerned with the welfare of the individual patient that, at times, the needs of society seem scarcely to be acknowledged. On the other hand, much of the lawyer's time must be taken up with balancing the respective claims of society and the individual; and at times the needs of the individual must seem of small importance besides the over-riding demands of the law of the land. The problem becomes more involved when the person under judicial examination is mentally ill. The psychiatrist must, by his training and outlook, come to see the offender as a sick man in need of treatment, whereas the judge, as the representative of society, may well only see him as a criminal requiring a long period of detention for the protection of others. Between these two extreme points of view it is necessary to reach a mutual understanding so that neither society, which has a right to be protected, nor the individual, who has a right to be treated, should be wholly excluded from consideration in the interests of one side or the other. So long as exclusive claims are made, then so long will the situation be strained.[4]

Exclusive claims are made by sovereigns as well as by disciplines. During the long history of the struggles of neighbor against neighbor, two sides have laid claims to many border areas. This is debatable land, defined by Webster as "a tract of land the ownership of which is in dispute between the two countries."

Law has jurisdiction over its own territory; psychiatry rules firmly in its area. Between them lies the debatable land, claimed by both but with neither in command. Like the best known of debatable lands, the tract between the Esk and Sark that was "claimed by both England and Scotland, and for a long time the subject of dispute," it is an area of bogs and mists and hidden dangers, "the haunt of thieves and vagabonds."[5] When the traveler is safely beyond the Esk or the Sark, he proceeds through well-regulated territory, but behind him, in the debatable land, two sides still face each other, sometimes asserting their exclusive claims, sometimes ready to find common solutions.

There is a realm of law, where the emphasis is on logic, and there is a domain of psychiatry, where feeling holds sway. At their border lie uncertainties and confusion. To the extent that psychiatry and law may find grounds for agreement, order is brought to the debatable land.

CHAPTER 2

The Point of View of Law

ALTHOUGH LAW and psychiatry have their differences, an individual is to be dealt with whose problems lie in the area where law and psychiatry meet, and whether he is called patient by the psychiatrist or client by the lawyer, the services of each may be called on. Psychiatry may say that it is in the best interest of the individual for him to be locked up in an institution against his will; the law will determine whether the psychiatrist or the patient will prevail. Law says the client cannot write a valid will or enter into a contract, or marry or divorce, because he does not have the mental capacity to do these things; but then the psychiatrist must examine the client to see whether the lawyer's opinion agrees with medical opinion. Whether a patient has the right to vote, or drive a car, or send mail, or practice his profession is an area where the lawyer and the psychiatrist—often the superintendent of the hospital where the patient has been committed—become mutually involved.

The relationship of the two disciplines is sometimes strained. It can be less strained if lawyers learn to look at some things in the way that psychiatrists do, and if psychiatrists learn to look at some things in the light of the legal tradition.

MAIN LEGAL THEMES

From the point of view of law, psychiatrists might bring to the mutual problem the understanding that certain themes appear and reappear through all branches of law. Some of these themes have come down from the early days of the Anglo-Saxon formulation of law and have spread into all the areas of today's law; others have been worked out by the courts in more recent times but nevertheless are universally accepted. The same themes are found in the subjects of contracts and wills, domestic relations and crime, consent and commitment, as well as the other areas of concern to forensic psychiatry. By tracing them, we can outline a unified system that underlies legal decisions, although the unity is often obscured by surface confusions and conflicts.

SANCTITY OF CONTRACT

The first of these themes, developed in English law over long centuries, is the sanctity of the contract. In the Middle Ages, promises were binding only if certain forms were observed or if they fell within the scope of statutes or previous decisions. Gradually, the courts became willing to enforce more and more mutual promises and agreements as contracts, both because the growing needs of mercantilism demanded strong legal backing of business arrangements, and because the mutual trust that made possible increasingly complex relationships between people was not possible under a system where one could evade the effect of his agreement by pleading a technicality, such as by saying that a promise to buy land was not under seal. By the late 1800s, English jurists saw the contract as sacred, the cornerstone of society. Wrote one eminent judge in an 1875 opinion: "if there is one thing more than another which public policy requires, it is that men of full age and competent understanding shall have the utmost liberty of contracting and that their contracts, when entered into freely and voluntarily, shall be held sacred and shall be enforced by courts of justice."[1] And a few years later Henry Sidgwick wrote in his *Elements of Politics:* "Suppose contracts freely made and effectively sanctioned, and the most elaborate social organisation becomes possible, at least in a society of such human beings as the individualistic theory contemplates—gifted with mature reason and governed by enlightened self-interest."[2]

Yet even though the contract is sacred in modern English law, the courts will uphold it only if certain requirements are met. It must not be against public policy; the courts will not enforce a contract to perform an illegal act.

SPECIAL PROTECTION

The contracting parties should have some equality of status. This brings us to a second theme. The law has always given special protection to the unfortunate and the helpless. Society has long recognized the need to protect the young, the deranged, the blind, the illiterate. Widows and orphans have been given special consideration by the law, and so have married women and seamen, the former two because they were weak and the latter two because they were under the domination of an authority, husband or captain, who could interfere with their pursuit of legal remedies. Wives have now been given substantially the same status as other contracting parties, but minors, seamen, and the mentally disabled find themselves in the common position of having fewer rights than the average citizen, but also of having greater protection from the courts.

The courts will try to protect the unfortunate; they will depart from their neutral position and lean over backwards to help. Particularly when the unfortunate is that least able of all mankind to protect his legal interests—when he is a dead testator who is no longer around to see that the provisions of his will are faithfully carried out—the law will do its best to try to carry out the testator's wishes whether he was sane or insane when the will was written.

CONSENT AND INTENT

A third theme that runs through all phases of the law is the importance of consent and intention. The law has sanctified the contract, but before it tries to enforce it, it must be sure that there *is* a contract.

Many of the early English cases revolve around the issue of whether a contract has really come into being, because before a contract can exist there must be a "meeting of the minds," a real understanding between the contracting parties about the gist of the contract. Many of the old cases involve agreements to buy and sell land. Farmer A wants to buy three acres of bottom land from Farmer B and offers him $100 an acre. He has in mind the pasture that borders on his own land. Farmer B agrees to the sale, but he plans to deed three other acres. There is no contract because there is no "meeting of the minds." Now, if the contract has been set down on paper and described in surveyors' language, and if both farmers have affixed their seals or gone through some such formality to show that they are solemnly entering into a formal contract, the words of the contract will take precedence. Farmer A cannot say, "I thought I was buying three acres adjoining my land," because the contract specifically states that the land is bounded on the South by a line from the big elm tree to Old York Road. When he signed the contract he was expressing his intent, and since the document is unambiguous, his intent is presumed to be equally so. But if the contract is not reduced to a written description, or if the description is ambiguous (there may be two big elm trees), the court can then deal with the question of whether there has been a meeting of the minds.

If Farmer A is hallucinating or Farmer B thinks that he is the King of France, the question of when and where minds meet and what parts of minds do the meeting becomes more complicated. Even the fact that their document spells out the contract in concrete unambiguous terms does not prove that there was a real "meeting of the minds," and without this their contract is not valid.

The same theme with a slightly different emphasis is embodied in criminal law. Just as a meeting of the minds underlies the concept of the contract, intent is an essential aspect of most crimes. The criminal must intend to do his acts. If a somnambulist robs in his sleep, he is not necessarily a criminal; it is only if the prosecution can prove that he intended to rob while asleep that he can be found guilty of criminal wrongdoing.

The concept of consent before a bargain becomes binding and its counterpart in criminal law, *mens rea* (being of a mind to do the act; either intent to commit the act or negligence which results in certain harms) do not go so far back in English law as many other basic concepts. The early common law concerning torts—civil wrongs other than breach of contract for which damages may be sought—held the defendant liable for accidental injuries that were unintended and took little or no account of his motives. It was only by a slow process and at a later date that such justification as self-defense was recognized.[3]

Toward the close of the nineteenth century, according to Prosser, the law had moved so far in the direction of looking into motives that some writers attempted to construct a consistent theory of tort law on the principle that there should be no liability without "blame." Today courts will look into motives in some cases, such as a case involving malicious prosecution or the building of a spite fence; in some other situations, such as the responsibility of an employer for accidents befalling his workmen, motive, intent and fault are not material.[4] But the latter type of situation represents a modern exception to our common law emphasis on liability as a result of blame and blame involving a particular state of mind.

INDIVIDUAL RIGHTS

The fourth theme is the protection of individual rights. Of all rights, freedom of movement, the freedom to come and go as one wills, is perhaps the most important. Forensic psychiatry is an area where rights and liberties may be denied; people who otherwise could vote or drive a car or marry or beget children or move about in freedom are deprived of any or all of these possibilities because they are considered and adjudged to be mentally ill. Virginia Woolf, who knew as a patient how restrictive the pronouncements of a psychiatrist can be, has described the effect of a fictional psychiatrist, Sir William Bradshaw, on the mentally ill who cross his professional path:

To his patients he gave three-quarters of an hour; and if in this exacting science which has to do with what, after all, we know nothing about—the nervous system, the human brain—a doctor loses his sense of proportion, as a doctor he fails. Health we must have; and health is proportion; so that when a man comes into your room and says he is Christ (a common delusion), and has a message, as they mostly have, and threatens, as they often do, to kill himself, you invoke proportion; order rest in bed; rest in solitude; silence and rest; rest without friends, without books, without messages; six months' rest; until a man who went in weighing seven stone six comes out weighing twelve.

Proportion, divine proportion, Sir William's goddess, was acquired by Sir William walking hospitals, catching salmon, begetting one son in Harley Street by Lady Bradshaw, who caught salmon herself and took photographs scarcely to be distinguished from the work of professionals. Worshipping proportion, Sir William not only prospered himself but made England prosper, secluded her lunatics, forbade childbirth, penalised despair, made it impossible for the unfit to propagate their views until they, too, shared his sense of proportion. . . .[5]

But if the law protects the unfortunate, our second theme, it also is jealous of liberty and conservative in dealing with human rights. The law will say to psychiatric patients, as it says to no other class in our society: Although you have done no wrong and are not a criminal, we will lock you up for an indeterminate period of time and take away your rights in very much the same manner that we do when we deal with criminals. The law is willing to go to this extreme, but it does so with due recognition that it is going to an extreme. Because the law takes away rights, it must scrutinize every phase of the process by which these rights are divested. So the protection of the rights of the mentally disabled becomes, for us, perhaps the paramount theme in the fabric of psychiatric law.

CHAPTER 3

The Point of View of Psychiatry

WHAT PSYCHIATRY is we have not said, although we have spoken a brief word about law and psychiatry. To complicate the matter, we have to consider not one psychiatry but at least two, possibly more.

Psychiatry is the portion of medical science that diagnoses and treats mental disease and cares for the mentally ill. It has been with us a long time. Doctors of medicine, sometimes called psychiatrists or alienists, have for centuries guarded and dosed mental patients, twirled them in revolving chairs, chained them to walls, freed them from their chains, prescribed rest and tranquility, prescribed activity and change, and even fired off cannons in the hope that the disease would be shocked out of existence. More recently, this same medical science has advocated removal of the appendix, of part of the bowel, even of part of the connections of the frontal lobes of the brain, in order to cure patients.

This type of psychiatry, whether we are speaking of a century ago or now, has always been interested in categorizing, classifying, putting names to conditions—nosology. True, many of the names do not survive the test of time, and some are popular in one part of the globe and not in another. Many of the patients we now consider schizophrenic, borderline psychotics, or sociopaths—and there can be arguments about what these terms really mean—were once labeled "constitutional inferiors," on the theory that defective germ plasm, descended from their progenitors, had biologically produced the sad specimens presented to us. Whether these cases have a biologic basis is not now and perhaps never will be known, but in the meantime, the term is out of fashion in this country, although still popular in other parts of the world. So, too, is the concept, which developed in Italy, of criminal types whose biologic inheritance—revealed in such stigmata as the shape of the ear lobes—determined that they would lead a life of crime. This concept has been popular at some times and in some places, but the feeling grows that the scientific assurance that earlier psychiatrists attributed to such theories and nosological schemes was not really scientific after all.

NEUROPSYCHIATRY

The type of psychiatry that is nosological and empirical has its modern counterpart in the neuropsychiatrist or, as he is sometimes called, the organicist. These names are not generally used; when a psychiatrist takes the witness stand, he identifies himself as a psychiatrist, not as a neuropsychiatrist. Courts have not recognized that these psychiatrists, lineal descendants of the alienist, are not interested in the unconscious factors that underlie an emotional state or an action.

The neuropsychiatrist is not a neurologist; he is a psychiatrist like any other doctor who, after internship, completes a three-year residency in psychiatry. But his point of view is bounded by neuroanatomy, neurophysiology, and psychopharmacology; he does not see the individual as in a state of conflict caused by opposing psychic forces. Psychiatrists differentiate this kind of psychiatrist from the other large school of modern psychiatrists by describing him as nondynamic or nonanalytic, or sometimes even as antianalytic.

To this psychiatrist, writes Karl Lewin, symptoms are synonymous with illness, and symptomatic relief is the goal of treatment.[1]

Although he may be aware that an unconscious exists, he does not feel that unconscious conflicts cause symptoms, nor does he view emotional illness as a recurrence of an infantile neurosis. The interpretation of dreams is not an essential part of treatment. Most important, the patient-doctor relationship (transference) is not analyzed. Instead, the neuropsychiatrist deals actively with the patient in his current life situation, giving advice, quite directively, and often dispensing medications. Frequently, he manipulates the patient's environment, or uses a special device such as hypnosis, electroshock treatment, or deconditioning. The neuropsychiatric approach is exhortative, directive, and repressive.

Hodern has stated that the neuropsychiatric or organic approach is empirical and continues to make fruitful contributions to psychiatric treatment and research; he feels that in spite of the fact that nondynamic psychiatrists are sometimes considered blind to emotional aspects of psychiatric disease, this approach in the best hands is not narrow or limited.[2]

DYNAMIC PSYCHIATRY

The second type of psychiatry may be called medical psychology, and it owes its beginnings largely to Sigmund Freud. It makes a difference whether you consult a non-Freudian or a Freudian psychiatrist. The former will have many patients in his waiting room, see patients for short periods of time, and may recommend drugs, electric shock or, in an extremity, psychosurgery; the latter will have few patients in his waiting room, will probably see each patient for a forty-five or fifty minute period, and will instruct many of his patients to lie on his couch and say whatever comes to mind.

The Freudian psychiatry has been called dynamic psychiatry, because it is interested in the equilibrium and the stresses on that equilibrium that exist among the theoretically formulated structures and layers of the mind. Dynamics in physical science has been defined as the branch of physics that deals with force as producing or affecting motion. Dynamics in medical psychology deals with forces in humans that produce or affect emotion and, subsequently, actions.

Dynamic psychiatry deals with two layers of the mind, the *conscious* and the *unconscious;* three structures of the mind, the *Id*, the *Ego* and the *Superego;* two main drives, *love* and *aggression*; and a multitude of *defensive ways* that are used to balance these factors so that the individual maintains a homeostatic equilibrium. Some of these defenses have been given labels: *isolation, denial, regression, sublimation, rationalization* and many more. The modern dynamic psychiatrist has as his task the *breaching of these defenses* when they are used to excess, i.e., pathologically, so that the original impulses that led to the development of the defenses can be understood and dealt with.

DIFFERENCE OF OPINION

Now, to add to the problem, most psychiatrists are neither clearcut non-Freudians who are interested in classifying, or clearcut Freudians who are interested in a verbal treatment; in most modern psychiatrists there is a mixture of both points of view. But usually one side or the other predominates. Take the case of the malingerer. To make the issue clearcut, let us assume that Private Jones has been heard to say: "No one can keep me in this man's army. All you have to do to get a discharge is to pretend you're a psycho." He later turns up on sick call with a full complement of psychiatric symptoms. The non-Freudian approach might be: This man is a malingerer, trying to deceive; he is therefore a bad character; perhaps a term in the jailhouse would help him see the error of his ways and, even if it doesn't, it would be appropriate punishment. The dynamic psychiatrist might say: A normal person wants to survive Army service with a good record and self-respect, and even though this man is pretending to have an emotional illness, he would not be pretending if in fact he were not emotionally ill; an investigation into his early years might show us why his male identifications are so lacking: an honorable discharge, based on psychoneurotic criteria, would be appropriate.

To add to the further complexity of the problem, the average psychiatrist probably cannot come to a clear-cut decision on this soldier. Part of his tradition is Freudian, part non-Freudian; he uses diagnostic terminology borrowed from one school and formulations borrowed from another; and when he is on the witness stand, he finds himself presenting ambiguous and vaguely thought-out points of view as if they were scientific facts. So we find in our courts of law, where adversary procedure is supreme, the spectacle that psychiatrist contradicts psychiatrist, and judges ask in vain for one definite opinion of the diagnosis and the prognosis of the defendant.

In any law proceeding, two adversary witnesses can come to different conclusions and testify accordingly. One expert may testify that it is standard medical procedure to perform a cesarean section or a radical mastectomy or to put a leg in traction under a given set of circumstances. But at least they can come to a common agreement about the patient's basic condition.

Only in forensic psychiatry, perhaps, can a psychiatrist, testifying in defense of an adolescent who murdered his father, state that the defendant was suffering from a *cyclothymic crisis*, during which impulses otherwise resistible now become irresistible, and thus persuade a jury to acquit the defendant—despite the fact that most psychiatric texts have never used the term *cyclothymic crisis* and that most psychiatrists cannot define it. And only in forensic psychiatry can a psychiatrist testify that an adult male who sexually assaulted a minor child is readily amenable to treatment and would have a good prognosis if, instead of being jailed, he were remanded to the custody of the psychiatrist for psychotherapy, and on that basis be awarded custody of the accused for continued psychotherapy—despite the fact that most psychiatrists would consider the accused not readily amenable to treatment.

Just as some judges see things from the point of view of the dynamic psychiatrist, and "naively" expect the psychiatrist to "cure the psychopath in ten easy lessons . . . secure in the belief that the probing of mischief in the unconscious would quickly solve all the problems of their clientele,"[3] some psychiatrists see things from the lawyer's traditional point of view. Dr. Robert Jones, Professor of Psychiatry at Dalhousie University, Halifax, was a member of the Royal Commission appointed by the government of Canada to inquire into the law of insanity as a defense in criminal cases. After two years of hearing testimony from lawyers and psychiatrists throughout Canada, he observed:

My experience in listening to psychiatric testimony across the country made me feel that some of my colleagues who had spent a good part of their professional life in contact with the psychopathic criminal had indeed developed very much the same kind of feelings as many lawyers. I would suggest that ... the attitudes of both professions are not determined entirely by their early training but are modified by their day-to-day experience. Lawyers are not always tough, demanding vengeance; psychiatrists are not always merciful with the feeling that everyone should be treated and no one should be punished. There are hanging judges, and there are hanging psychiatrists. On a number of occasions, psychiatrists who devoted a good deal of their professional life to the examination of criminals, and who usually appeared for the prosecution in any such trials that happen in a particular geographical area, frequently seemed to have lost their "therapeutic orientation" and had it replaced by a "punishment orientation."[4]

When psychiatric experts disagree, the fault may easily be made to appear psychiatry's, and a court may conclude that all psychiatry is to blame. But in psychiatry, as in any other discipline, there are necessarily conflicting views and there are areas of backwardness, stupidity, even venality. The blame for the resulting confusion is easily placed on the conflicting experts. The judiciary may sit high above the conflict and, without taking the time or trouble to learn much about modern psychiatric thought, will sometimes use the difference in expert opinion to secure the legal result it desires and then to call down the psychiatrists for the confusion they have brought into the courtroom.

CHAPTER 4

Psychiatrist in Court

L AW AND PSYCHIATRY start from different premises, have different purposes and points of view. To the psychiatrist, one additional fact basic to the legal system is unsettling: the Anglo-Saxon system of justice is an adversary system. That implies that the two contestants meet in court as they met in battle in earlier days. Each adversary presents to the court not the true picture of his case but, instead, his strongest case; and the court and the jury will have the task of sifting through the evidence for the kernel of actuality.

ADVERSARY SYSTEM

The two adversaries (plaintiff vs defendant or, in a criminal case, State vs accused) have at issue a difference of opinion concerning law or the facts of the case—or, and this is usual, differences of both fact and law. The differences of law are argued before the court; the judge, and the judges of superior courts who may review the case, are the final arbiters. The differences of fact are argued before the jury; twelve impartial (hopefully) men, after hearing the stories of both sides, decide what, in the light of the evidence they have heard, may fairly be taken to be the facts.

I may argue that I did not steal your pumpkins and, even if I did (for no one has ever said that pleas must be consistent), their monetary value was so slight that the case does not come within the scope of the legislation cited by the prosecution. Whether the case has been brought properly is a matter for the judge; when he has decided that the action has been properly brought, it is the turn of the jury to listen to evidence concerning factual matters—I present witnesses who say I was in another county on the night concerned; the prosecution presents witnesses who saw me fleeing from the scene—and then to decide which witness is most to be believed.

Now, because we are working in the framework of an adversary system, some corollaries will necessarily follow.

One, each side will be represented by the best obtainable attorneys, and these attorneys will do their utmost to discredit the witnesses of the opposing

26

side, even though privately they may have no doubt of the truth of the testimony of the opposing witnesses.

Two, each side will secure the services of the best obtainable experts, and these experts will also face the cross-examination and the attempt to discredit them by the attorney of the opposing side.

Three, despite the fact that experts have appeared, a jury composed of nonexperts will have the final decision which expert is most to be believed.

This is a state of affairs that doctors, who tend to be authoritarian and who often take themselves and their own opinions seriously, find deplorable. Many of the proposals of recent years—that technical matters concerning sanity, medical diagnoses, and other medical matters be removed from the arena of the adversary procedure and put into the hands of a panel or group of experts acting as consultants to the court—have their origin in the wounded vanity of medical experts. Those who push hardest to remove much of the subject of the trial from the trial procedure are often those least aware of the protection to individual liberties that is the product of the adversary system, and the least knowledgeable about the long history of hardfought victories that has culminated in the unwieldy and inefficient system of justice, which, in spite of all its drawbacks, deserves such praise as that of Lewis: "Civilization has yet to produce a better system of adjudicating the differences between man and man, and man and institution, than the Anglo-Saxon administration of law."[1]

WEIGHT OF PSYCHIATRIC TESTIMONY

Dr. Samuel Woodhouse, of Pennsylvania, in 1953 murdered his adolescent adopted daughter in her sleep. She suffered from a progressive neurologic disease; the doctor, according to testimony at his trial, felt that he had an incurable disease (he did not) and that his daughter's condition would inevitably deteriorate. He foresaw that his wife would be left to cope with an unmanageable situation at so me point in the future. He tried to kill his daughter by shooting her in the head with a rifle in her third floor bedroom, then returned to his office on the ground floor where he treated two patients. Later, finding his daughter unconscious but not dead, he administered a dose of methadone and then gave himself a presumably fatal injection of the same drug. He was discovered unconscious.

The doctor was adjudged insane and not able to stand trial. He spent the next four years in state mental hospitals. Then, adjudged cured by the hospital staff, he was tried for murder in the first degree. Eminent psychiatrists, two of them imported from Philadelphia for the occasion, who had examined him in the months following the murder, testified that he had always been obsessive and unstable. Witnesses were presented to demonstrate a history of personality change ante-dating the crime by at least a year—unhappiness, irritability, morose-ness, lack of memory, worries about his health, his daughter's health and her antisocial attitude. Evidence presented included the finding of the lunacy commission shortly after the crime that he was insane, the testimony of a state psychiatrist that he suffered from paranoid schizophrenia, and the testimony of both a psychiatrist for the defense and an impartial psychiatrist that he had suffered from a paranoid involutional psychosis.

No psychiatric testimony rebutted the unanimous testimony of the experts that the doctor was not only insane at the time of the murder but also unable to appreciate fully the nature and quality of his act, thus bringing the case under the M'Naghten doctrine, the basis of the defense. Opposed to the testimony of the experts, however, was the testimony of neighbors and patients who had seen the doctor on the day of the murder, been treated by him with his usual medical thor-oughness, and could report that he did not seem different from his usual self. A report on his state of mind at the time of his arrest by police authorities said "the physician showed no remorse for the crime, worked in his garden after the slaying and treated two patients while the girl lay dead in the house."

In his instruction to the jury, the judge said: "You will consider the opinions of the psychiatrists. You must consider their training, qualifications and experience, and the date or dates when they examined the defendant. It must be kept in mind that an opinion is only an opinion. It creates no fact. Because of this, opinion evidence is con-sidered of low grade and not entitled to much weight against positive testimony of actual facts such as statements by the defendant and observations of his actions."

The jury found the defendant guilty of first degree murder, thus giving no weight to the uncontradicted expert testimony. This de-cision was affirmed by the Pennsylvania Supreme Court:[2]

The lay witnesses called by the Commonwealth in rebuttal testified to *actual facts*. The executive officer of the Boy Scouts and the young lady patient, who saw the defendant on the same morning, right after the murder, had the unusual opportunity of seeing and observing him at a most important hour. Even witnesses called by the defense testified as to the normal conduct of the defendant on the day of the killing. They testified as to what they saw. . . . Actual facts, proven by positive evidence, are under the law of Pennsylvania entitled to far more weight than opinion evidence, even that of experts.

The court does not seem to have given consideration to the fact that normal behavior under these circumstances is abnormal indeed.

In his dissent, Justice Musmanno defended psychiatric testimony.

The evidence of doctors in a case of this kind is not "low grade." They have studied and they have been trained to analyze mental disorders. They have had many years of experience, they have seen and analyzed hundreds of cases. They are certainly in a far better position to diagnose a mental illness than a casual observer. . . .

The jury had the right to be assisted in the discharge of their awesome duties by listening to doctors who have dedicated their lives to determining the why and wherefore of the inexplicable. But when the Judge told the jury that the testimony of the three physicians was "low grade," he practically wiped it out of the case and when he did this he deprived the defendant of a fair trial.

Cases like this, in which the weight of psychiatric testimony is disregarded, concern psychiatrists. Having taken a minimum three-year residency in their specialty, following four years of medicine, psychiatrists would prefer the court to accept their word about whether a person is sane or insane, competent or incompetent. They believe that psychiatric testimony should be given more weight than that of a nonexpert, and feel that a crowning indignity is that the twelve men on the jury, who may not know a chronic ambulatory schizophrenic from a Ganser's syndrome, determine questions technical and psychiatric.

WEIGHT OF MEDICAL TESTIMONY

Other physicians, not psychiatrists, have the same problem in court; they would like to see their testimony on mental capacity treated as conclusive. But the courts continue to treat it merely as testimony to be weighed against other contradictory testimony in the formulation of a decision. A recent Illinois case concerned a suit to set aside a will on the ground that the testator had been under undue influence and did not have the mental capacity to make a valid will. The testator had suffered a stroke after executing the will, and the intern from the hospital to which she had been taken and her family physician both testified that she was senile and lacked mental capacity to make a will. On the opposing side, three witnesses, not physicians, testified that in their opinion the testator did have the necessary mental capacity. The lawyer seeking to have the will declared valid asked that one of the judge's instructions to the jury be the following: "Although physicians are better qualified to testify to a diseased condition than laymen, their testimony upon the subject of the mental capacity of an individual . . . is not entitled to any greater weight than that of laymen." The judge felt this instruction was improper and refused so to instruct the jury, but on appeal the Illinois Supreme Court has ruled that the requested instruction was proper.[3]

WEIGHT OF PSYCHOLOGICAL TESTIMONY

Not only is the medical and psychiatric witness not given the consideration in court that he may feel he deserves, and not only is testimony of nonexpert witnesses given equal weight in the determination of mental capacity in some cases but even more alarming to the psychiatrist, the psychologist in some courts is considered his equal as an expert witness. In the District of Columbia case of *Jenkins* vs *United States*, the American Psychiatric Association felt so strongly about this matter that it filed a brief contending:

> The psychologist, not being a qualified Doctor of Medicine, with special training in the care and treatment of the mentally ill, in our view, cannot qualify as a medical expert in the diagnosis, treatment and care of the mentally ill. The unique qualifications of the trained psychiatrist qualify him as the expert on the medical aspects of diseases of the mind. The psychiatrist's diagnosis of mental illnesses should be based on the *synthesis* of data from several sources. Psychological tests are but a part of the problem, and the clinical psychologist administering such tests is not qualified to ultimately diagnose a specific mental illness or defect or give expert medical testimony as to the existence of a special mental disease or specific mental defect. . . .

The majority opinion, written by Judge Bazelon (famous as the author of the *Monte Durham* decision regarding criminal responsibility) for the US Court of Appeals, stated that some psychologists are qualified to testify concerning diagnosis and treatment of mental disease or defect and that the determination of a psychologist's competence "to render an expert opinion based on his findings as to the presence or absence of mental disease or defect must depend upon the nature and extent of his knowledge. It does not depend on his claim to the title 'psychologist.' And that determination, after hearing, must be left in each case to the traditional discretion of the trial court. . . ."[4]

IMPARTIAL EXPERTS

More and more, the plea is made that questions of insanity and mental capacity be taken out of the adversary phase of a trial and reserved for a behind-the-scene determination where, without the intrusion of a jury, men of science can speak their pieces and make their determinations without fear of contradiction or rejection. Even some judges, tired of hearing experts on opposing sides give completely different answers to the famous lengthy hypothetical questions, sometimes look with favor on a system where impartial experts behind the scene will predetermine some issues of fact that up to this time have been left for jury determination.

One typical proposal, put forward with vehemence by a psychiatrist, asks for an impartial examination of the accused before trial and "preferably before arraignment," when the issue of insanity has not yet been raised. Another part of this same proposal is the avoidance of the use of the resulting impartial medical testimony until after the guilt or innocence is determined: "After this verdict is in, *and only then*, competent medical testimony can be introduced to aid the judge in the determination of sentencing and the proper disposition of the case."[5]

This psychiatrist is guilty of a fault common to both lawyer and psychiatrist, of furnishing easy answers to hard questions. In the first place, impartiality is not secured by the fact of court appointment. Says Henry Davidson: "I am doubtful about court-appointed experts. If the jury does not know that the doctor is court-appointed, there is no point in the system. If the jury *does* know it, then this doctor invisibly wears the robe of a judge and the halo of a saint. . . . no human being can be impartial: we must identify with one side or the other, the identification being based on our personal background and prejudices."[6] Another point raised by Davidson: ". . . in psychiatry, nothing is 100 per cent. Whether a person has a simple schizophrenia or a schizoid personality, it is not a matter of true or false. It seems to me that the adversary system is the honest way of exposing the truth. The expert who thinks it is a psychosis has his say and explains why; the other expert does the same. Truth has many sides and the system of having each side present its own expert is one way of showing that."[7]

The drastic proposals to remove psychiatric questions from the courtroom overlook the fact that justice as it has developed gives the accused, among others, the following rights:

To obtain for himself the expert whom he trusts most.

To challenge the competency of the opposition expert.

To have the court hear both sides.

To have the element of intent or *mens rea*, when an essential part of a crime, proved by the prosecution.

To have a choice of pleading insanity or not as his own best interest indicates.

To be free from enforced psychiatric examination before arraignment, when no crime is charged.

To have conflicting opinions made a matter of public record, so that they can be considered by a superior court on appeal and brought to the attention of the public through the press.

To have a conviction based on the opinion of a jury.
To have the advantage of a presumption of innocence.
To prevent the deification of a single point of view.

In more subjective terms, Canada's Dr. Robert Jones has said:
"I would hesitate to leave my fate, were I found guilty of murder, in
the hands of some of my professional brethren who have spent 30 years
testifying as crown witnesses. Experts can be exceedingly biased. I
would believe that justice is more likely to result from the deliberation
of 12 good men and true, who, though ignorant, are able to empathize
with the man in the dock, than from the deliberations of many of the
individuals who would form the majority of a panel of experts."[8]

The *Report of the American Bar Foundation*, in its section dealing
with the laws regarding the involuntary hospitalization of sexual psychopaths, deals with the question of the relationship between the
opinions of experts and legal safeguards:

> The difficulty in establishing a legal definition and descriptive criteria
> within sexual psychopath legislation has resulted in a transfer of responsibility
> from the legal trier of fact to the psychiatric expert. The vague criteria give
> the expert extremely wide latitude as to who may be called a deviate. The
> question is raised whether in such a case the power of hospitalization has been
> transferred to the medical witness. Although the statutes require the court to
> listen to testimony generally, traditions have developed whereby the finding
> of psychopathy by the medical expert is sufficient for hospitalization. In light
> of the indeterminate sentence and the criminal aspects of the proceedings,
> careful consideration must be given to the consequences of such a transfer of
> responsibility. It even has been suggested that the jury in the hospitalization
> proceedings be replaced by a panel of experts or that the entire proceedings take
> place before a commission of experts. The medical expert is not the proper
> person to determine whether an individual should be indeterminately hospital-
> ized against his will. The doctor does not always have the patient's individual
> rights in mind. The training of a lawyer focuses his attention on individual
> rights, privileges, and liberties. Consequently, a lawyer is more apt to regard
> these rights as foremost and all other considerations as secondary. A doctor,
> on the other hand, is trained to consider the patient's health as the primary
> factor.[9]

Those who wish to take the determination of sanity or mental
capacity out of the adversary procedure arena overlook the fact that
the jury system was brought into being to safeguard the rights of the
individual, that it acts in criminal cases (since a unanimous decision is
customarily required for conviction) to weight the balance in favor of
the defendant, which is in accordance with our view that innocence is
presumed, and that the so-called scientific classification in modern psychiatry has almost as many detractors as it has adherents. They over-

look the fact that when matters heretofore determined by jury are
allowed to be decided by a board or panel of so-called experts, the
individual before the bar has lost some portion of his civil rights. To
the lawyer, it seems important that civil rights be preserved; to the
psychiatrist, who believes that his diagnosis or prognosis should be
accepted without challenge, these rights seem less important.

Concerning Contracts

THE ENGLISH LAW on contracts, from which American law is derived, is based largely on the concept of mutual assent. Before a contract is considered validly begun, a mutual obligation must be formulated and both parties must assent to its terms. Each party has an understanding about what the terms under discussion really mean. The phrase "meeting of the minds" has been used to describe the mutual agreement that a contract puts into formal terms.

Still, a contract may sometimes result even though the minds do not actually meet—as when, despite a discrepancy between the intentions of the two contracting parties, they enter into a contract so unambiguous that it would indicate to an objective third party that an agreement really has been ratified. Judge Learned Hand has dealt with the notion that a contracting party's idiosyncratic intention, rather than the sense of a written document, should prevail: "A contract has, strictly speaking, nothing to do with the personal, or individual, intent of the parties. A contract is an obligation attached by the mere force of law to certain acts of the parties, usually words which ordinarily accompany and represent a known intent."[1] Other opinions can be cited for the same proposition:

A contract involves what is called a meeting of the minds of the parties. But this does not mean that they must have arrived at a common mental state touching the matter at hand. The standard by which their conduct is judged and their rights are limited is not internal, but external. In the absence of fraud or incapacity, the question is: "What did the party say and do? "The making of a contract does not depend upon the state of the parties' mind; it depends on their overt acts."[2]

But although the written document indicating a meeting of the minds may take precedence over the contracting party's statement that there was no mutual assent, the concept of mutual assent is fundamental to the law of contract. Defendant contracted to buy 125 bales of Surat cotton arriving on the ship *Peerless* from Bombay. When the cotton arrived, he refused to accept the goods because he said he had intended the contract to apply to goods arriving on the ship *Peerless* that sailed from Bombay in October; the goods had not arrived on this ship but on a ship, also named *Peerless*, which sailed from Bombay two months later.

The plaintiff in this 1864 case,[3] often cited for the proposition that there can be no contract without a "meeting of the minds," demanded that defendant accept the goods and pay for them: "the contract was for the sale of a number of bales of cotton of a particular description, which the plaintiff was ready to deliver. It is immaterial by which ship the cotton was to arrive, so that it was a ship called the *Peerless*. The words 'to arrive ex *Peerless*,' only mean that if the vessel is lost on the voyage, the contract is to be at an end. . . . The defendant has no right to contradict by parol evidence, a written contract good upon the face of it. He does not impute misrepresentation or fraud, but only says that he fancied the ship was a different one. Intention is of no avail, unless stated at the time of the contract."

But the court agreed with the argument of the defendant that the meeting of the minds, essential to the formation of a contract, had been absent: "there is nothing on the face of the contract to show that any particular ship called the *Peerless* was meant; but the moment it appears that two ships called the *Peerless* were about to sail from Bombay there is a latent ambiguity, and parol evidence may be given for the purpose of showing that the defendant meant one *Peerless* and the plaintiff another. That being so, there was no consensus ad idem, and therefore no binding contract."

Although the law has emphasized the sanctity of contractual obligations, the contracts of the mentally disabled are given special status for two reasons. First, the law protects those with special disabilities— this is one of the themes that appears in all law. Second, a strong possibility exists in any contractual agreement where one party is incompetent that there was no true "meeting of the minds," and the mutuality of assent is a dominating principle.

The attitude of the court towards the psychiatrically ill has developed from the attitude it has long held towards infants, who labor under such disabilities as the lack of the right to manage their own property or to sign leases and contracts, and who must seek permission from parent or guardian before carrying on many legal activities. This sometimes looks onerous, but there is a brighter side when the infant wishes to escape the effect of an agreement and so pleads his infancy.

The disabilities of infants are really privileges, which the law gives them, and which they may exercise for their own benefit, the object of the law being to secure infants from damaging themselves or their property by their own improvident acts or prevent them from being imposed on by the fraud of others. While the rights of infants are not superior, they are of greater concern to a court of equity than those of adults, and the rights of infants must be protected by the court, while adults must protect their own rights. Persons dealing with the infant must take notice of his privileges and disabilities.[4]

The legal philosophy relating to the psychiatrically ill is similar. One minor difference, interesting only historically, was that under early English common law one could not plead insanity in order to escape the obligations of an agreement—presumably on the theory that if one is competent enough to conduct his own legal defense he could not be really insane, and that if one has recovered from insanity, he cannot be trusted to recall his intention and state of mind while insane. But since a relative or guardian could plead the insanity, the defense was well recognized under the law.[5] The law as it has evolved is that "insanity may be pleaded or set up in avoidance of a civil act. However, the incapacity cannot be changed from a shield of protection into a weapon of offense."[6]

The insane person is differentiated in one important way from other classes of unfortunates in that his condition is not necessarily seen as continuous or permanent. "An insane person is not civilly dead." In many jurisdictions, a person who is legally insane can enter into a contract in a lucid interval when the mental disability is not operating; the contract could then be voided if the lucid interlude could not be proved, but the contract would not automatically be void. In other jurisdictions, the fact that a person has been declared to be legally insane—even though the adjudication may merely represent a legal statement of a prior time that does not conform with the actual state of mental competency at the time a contractual agreement was entered into—makes his legal agreements not merely potentially voidable but actually void.[7]

The law has long held that if someone supplies necessaries—food, clothing, shelter—to an insane person or his wife under a contract or an implied contract, the insanity is no defense against a claim for a reasonable reimbursement for the necessaries furnished.[8] But contracts covering other less ordinary transactions do come within the scope of the doctrine described, and the law will consider them voidable.

The enforceability of contracts presented less of a problem in earlier days, when patients were more clearly seen as either insane or recovered, than it does in a time when hospitals are used flexibly, when patients leave the hospital on shopping trips and weekend passes, or even work in the day and are hospital patients only at night. Psychiatrists have begun to abandon the former classifications, where health and disease are clearly demarcated, and now speak in terms of a spectrum ranging from the "normal" (that hypothetical construct) to the very regressed psychotic, with all stages of health and illness ranged in various degrees between the two extremes. Psychiatrists find increasing use for the concept of ego functions intact in some areas and lacking in others.

How does the law consider the patient whose illness is compartmentalized, restricted to only a few aspects of his functioning? "Although it was at one time considered," says *Corpus Juris Secundum*, "that a person afflicted only with an insane delusion, or insanity on some particular subject, was not capable of performing any civil act requiring volition, it is now well understood that a man may be thoroughly insane on one subject and at the same time be quite capable of transacting business on all others; and to void a man's act on the ground of insane delusion it is necessary to show that the act under judicial consideration was the direct result of such delusion."[9]

Do voluntary patients stand in a better position than involuntary as regards contractual competency? The law concerning the competency of the voluntary patient to conduct such business affairs as he wishes is unclear in most jurisdictions. Texas is the only state that by statute provides that both voluntary and involuntary hospitalized patients retain their competency. Three other states, Arizona, Delaware, and South Dakota, provide by statute that involuntary patients retain competency, and by implication it can be assumed that voluntary patients do also. Another three states, Illinois, Ohio, and Oklahoma, expressly provide that voluntary patients retain competency.[10] The *Draft Act Governing Hospitalization of the Mentally Ill*, issued in 1952 by the National Institutes of Mental Health as a model for states to follow in revising their statutes, proposes this wording:

> Subject to the general rules and regulations of the hospital and except to the extent that the head of the hospital determines that it is necessary for the medical welfare of the patient to impose restrictions, every patient shall be entitled . . . to exercise all civil rights, including the right to dispose of property, execute instruments, make purchases, enter contractual relationships, and vote, unless he has been adjudicated incompetent and has not been restored to legal capacity.[11]

Five states—Idaho, Missouri, New Mexico, Tennessee, and Utah —have adopted the civil rights provisions of the model draft act, and a sixth, Georgia, has adopted them partially. In these states, patients not adjudicated incompetent retain contractual capacity if hospital rules permit and the head of the hospital is not in opposition; the question remains as to the extent of the discretionary power of hospital and hospital head. Most other states have no statutory provisions expressly saving the contractual capacity or other civil rights of voluntary patients.[12]

In any case where a court upholds the contract of a mentally disabled person, voluntary or involuntary, the court will of course scrutinize the transaction. If the contract is not adverse to the patient's interests, and in the absence of contrary statutory provisions, courts will not hesitate to find a contract valid if the patient is not under guardianship and can demonstrate a reasonable degree of mental awareness and contact with reality, and a reasonably intact memory.

In most jurisdictions, either the law is not clear or it is specifically stated that hospitalized patients cannot enter into valid contracts. Some states explicitly and others implicitly merge the fact of hospitalization and the presumption or adjudication of incompetency in spite of agreement between lawyers and psychiatrists that a person may be in need of hospital treatment for a psychiatric condition and still be competent.[13] The law does not oppose psychiatric opinion, but on this topic, it lags far behind.

Marriage

MARRIAGE is a contract. For it to come into effect, courts have held, the parties marrying must have sufficient mental competency to understand the nature of the contract that they are entering into and to understand that they are in fact getting married. Therefore someone drugged or drunk, or psychotic or senile, who entered into a marriage not knowing what marriage was all about, or not knowing that this ceremony was a marriage ceremony, would have grounds for annulment—or the guardian looking after the interests of such a person would have grounds to start annulment action—based on this lack of understanding on the part of the bride or groom.

Miss Able wishes to marry Mr. Baker, but she knows that Mr. Baker does not want to marry her. She then asks Mr. Baker to participate in a "mock marriage." She persuades her clergyman to take part in the deception and secures a marriage license. Mr. Baker of course cannot be married without his assent.

Foiled in this attempt, Miss Able plies Mr. Baker with liquor, drives him to a state where there is no "waiting period" and props him up while a brief ceremony is performed before the justice of the peace. Mr. Baker awakes the next morning in unfamiliar surroundings, to be told that where before he was single he is now double. Not so; Mr. Baker can still assert that he was not conscious of what was going on, did not consent to the terms of the marriage contract, and no valid contract of marriage exists. But he can only make this statement if he flees from the scene without intimacy with Miss Able. If at this point, aware of the fact that Miss Able asserts that they were legally married the previous night and that he has no conscious recollection of the ceremony, he throws caution to the winds and engages in intercourse with Miss Able, the act of intercourse at the time of understanding links up, in some way which only lawyers understand, with the marriage undertaken without understanding, and the marriage comes into being and is in fact retroactively valid from the time of the ceremony.

Sometimes a difficult decision concerning marriage has to be made not by the prospective bride or groom but by the superintendent of

the mental hospital where the prospective bride or groom is a patient.
Let us assume that Miss Able is a borderline mental deficient with an
I Q of 78 and that because of her temper outbursts, attempts to run
away from home and flagrant promiscuity, she has been committed to
a state hospital. While she is a committed patient, the superintendent
of the hospital has the legal responsibility of seeing that she does not
enter into disadvantageous contracts, including a disadvantageous contract of marriage. While home on a weekend visit, Miss Able cohabits
with her long-time boyfriend, Mr. Baker, and in due course the staff
of the hospital discovers that she is pregnant. Mr. Baker says he loves
Miss Able and wants to marry her. The hospital staff learns that he
has completed only seven grades of schooling, is only intermittently
employed, and comes from a family with a long history of delinquency
and mental illness. Should the superintendent of the state hospital
allow Miss Able to enter into this marriage—this being very much her
own and her family's wish—or should he conclude that Miss Able does
not have sufficient competency to understand the marriage bargain?
However he decides, the superintendent, if he values his own skin, will
have in the patient's record a number of statements of other physicians
supporting his decision.

   Besides the general principles governing marriage of the mentally
disabled, many states have passed laws that specifically prohibit the
marriage of some people regardless of whether they have the competency to enter into a marriage contract. Two reasons are given for
such statutes: the first is to prevent the creation of a marriage when
one prospective partner lacks sufficient reason fully to understand the
nature of the contract (i.e., rather than dealing with the individual and
ascertaining whether he has competency, the fact that the individual
has been placed in a special category before the law automatically brings
into effect the prohibition against marriage). Some of the categories
set forth in various statutes are: idiots, insane, weak-minded, lunatics,
feeble-minded, imbeciles, persons incapable of contracting, and persons
of unsound mind. Delaware is an example of a state with an unusually
far-reaching statute that prohibits not only persons of unsound mind
from marrying but also narcotic addicts, habitual drunkards, and
persons who are or have been patients in an insane asylum; a legal
marriage may take place if a patient or ex-patient in an asylum files
with the clerk of peace a certificate signed by the institution's superintendent stating that he is fit to marry.

   The second reason for statutory prohibitions of marriage is eugenic
—to prevent the birth of children who may be constitutionally or en-
vironmentally handicapped. In Kansas, persons adjudicated incapaci-
tated cannot marry unless the woman who is in the marriage is 45

years or older. Virginia and Washington also allow such marriages, otherwise prohibited, if the woman is over 45; Nebraska, which prohibits marriage of a person adjudicated an imbecile, feeble-minded, or afflicted with hereditary insanity or epilepsy, makes an exception if the mentally disabled prospective partner is sterilized.[1] Seven states have no statutory provisions against marriage, but do allow annulment or divorce if it is shown that one partner lacked competency.

Most such statutes are ambiguous; many of them use such non-medical terms as weak-minded or lunatic, and often do not state whether hospitalized patients or other subclasses of the mentally disabled are encompassed by the prohibition. Psychiatrists question the legislation because, among other reasons, many mentally ill persons who do not seek help and who are not hospitalized, or treated or even diagnosed, may be more disabled mentally than the persons covered by these statutes.

States with statutory prohibitions against such marriages do little to enforce their laws. Twenty states have some enforcement machinery, and nineteen of them have criminal penalties for violation of the statute. Four states—Illinois, Kansas, North Carolina and North Dakota—make a certificate, an affidavit or a statement regarding the absence of prohibited mental conditions a condition for the issuance of a marriage license.[2] Deutsch, in *The Mentally Ill in America*, has said that all statutes to prevent the marriages of people with mental disability have "invariably proved worthless, chiefly because of the lack of adequate provision for the identification or diagnosis of the mental status of applicants for marriage licenses."[3]

Certainly the provisions of state laws putting epileptics in the same category as the feeble-minded and the insane for the purpose of preventing marriages or making marriages voidable, while probably not enforced recently to any extent, represent an affront to the feelings of epileptics that cuts deep and has no relationship to modern medical thought on this topic.

Lindman and McIntyre, editors of the American Bar Foundation study *The Mentally Disabled and the Law*, point out the inconsistency of the policy of those states that consider a marriage improper but instead of prohibiting the marriage allow it to take place with the remedy offered of annulment or divorce on the showing that a partner lacked competency.

The threat of a severed marriage is not an effective deterrent to one who is incapable of understanding the marriage relationship, nor is dissolution an effective enforcement measure when it is dependent upon the voluntary initiative of one of the parties to the disapproved relationship.

If the state actually wishes to control marriages that it considers unadvised, more direct action should be taken. The most effective method might be to check all applications for marriage licenses against a central record file for all incompetent and hospitalized persons. A further requirement of a physician's certificate stating the absence of the prohibited conditions before a license could be issued would act as a check on persons who are mentally disabled but who have not been so adjudicated. The right to a judicial determination of competency to marry, if there has been a denial of marriage license on the basis of a medical certificate, should guarantee adequate protection of individual rights.[4]

Whether the state, which has so much trouble controlling and enforcing conditions that it clearly has the duty to control and enforce, wants to take on additional responsibility for supervision of the marriage state is, although Lindman and McIntyre do not point this out, a potentially controversial question. Should "big government" increase its supervision of this intimate relationship? What are the standards that determine whether one understands the marriage relationship? What if the effect of prohibiting marriages leads to more living together of unmarried couples? The present state of the law, although admittedly disorderly, is flexible enough to prevent the marriage of those clearly of unsound mind without too much interference with the rest of the citizenry, who may or may not have had emotional or psychiatric problems.

CHAPTER 7

Divorce

FROM ONE point of view, marriage is a permanent obligation, explicit in the words of the marriage vow, "till death us do part." If a woman marries a man who thereafter gets cancer, or tuberculosis, or leprosy or amyotrophic lateral sclerosis, she cannot come into court to say that her husband is hospitalized or ill, that he may be hospitalized for years, and in any case is in no position to be a help to her now or in the foreseeable future, and that on these grounds the marriage should be dissolved.

If shortly after a marriage, a husband has a psychotic episode, believes he is being followed, becomes assaultive and abusive, and has to be put into a mental hospital, and if it turns out that he does not improve in the hospital and is finally diagnosed as a chronic paranoid schizophrenic, there are some people who would argue that divorces should be allowed. They see a parallel in the cases of some criminals who are given extremely long jail sentences or life terms; the spouse is in some cases allowed to divorce the prisoner even without other ground, such as adultery or cruelty, and even if the prisoner opposes the suit. The law looks at the hardship involved; its reasoning appears to be that the prisoner by committing a felony (and getting caught) has made himself unavailable to his wife and that this is a violation of the marriage contract. So too, some would argue that mental illness makes it impossible for mutuality to exist in the marriage contract.

In spite of the fact that the well spouses of hospitalized psychiatric patients may often want a divorce, and in fact may feel that they need a husband or a wife who is well and able either to support or to keep house for a family—the predicament of a husband with several children whose wife seems incurably ill is difficult to overstate—the law in the past has tended to feel otherwise. We have said that the law will try to uphold a contract, and marriage is a civil contract. We have said that the law will lean over backwards to try to protect the helpless, and a hospitalized patient is substantially helpless. Insanity has therefore been considered a bar to a suit for divorce. The general rule of law has been that even though a well spouse has seemingly valid grounds for

43

divorcing a mentally ill partner—evidence of desertion or adultery or acts of cruelty—the suit could be defeated by a showing that the partner was either mentally ill when the grounds for divorce came into being, or that the partner was presently mentally ill.

The reasoning behind these answers to a divorce action are: if such acts as desertion or adultery took place while the wife was of unsound mind, she lacked the capacity to assent to the doing of these acts or the will to prevent their commission; and if they occurred prior to the onset of the mental illness, the divorce proceeding could not take place because the wife who was now psychotic presumably lacked the mental capacity to determine for herself whether to defend the suit. In the event that she did decide to defend it, she could not conduct herself to present the strongest possible defense.*

Most states, particularly the most populous, have consistently denied divorce on the ground of mental disability until the past several decades, even if this denial caused a prolonged or permanent marriage of separated partners. The *Report of the American Bar Foundation* points out that Arkansas, in 1843, and Washington, in 1886, are variously given credit for being the first state to permit divorce for post-nuptial mental illness. By 1931, 13 states had such statutory provisions; by 1946, 26 states; and now 30 have.[1] It points out that while Sweden's law allowing a divorce for insanity goes back more than 100 years, the idea gained acceptance very slowly, both in Europe and here.[2]

But even though statutes in a majority of states now permit the mentally disabled to be divorced, the terms of the statutes and the protection given to the hospitalized spouse effectively prevent many divorces from being granted. The statutes that allow divorce require the condition to have persisted for at least two years (most states specify at least five), except for Utah, which sets no specific time. The great "catch" is that almost all of the statutes on the subject require that the condition be incurable and more than one-half require that this incurability be established by medical testimony.[3]

The term "incurable" has less application in psychiatry than in other fields of medicine. Some psychiatric conditions that are organic are certainly incurable. But many of these, such as mental deficiency, appear at birth or early in life, and these statutes apply only to post-

---

* When we come to discuss criminal responsibility, we will see these same themes running through the topic—a criminal is not guilty if he lacks the mental capacity to know what he is doing or, even if he has that capacity at the time of the commission of the crime, he cannot be brought to trial if in the period between the commission of the crime and the time of the trial he has become insane. He cannot be tried until he has recovered from the psychosis and can cooperate with his counsel in his defense.

nuptial mental illness, conditions of mental disability that develop after the marriage has taken place.

Since these statutes thus have no application to most hereditary organic conditions, which manifest themselves in childhood or adolescence, they cover only late-arising organic psychiatric conditions—such as Alzheimer's or Pick's diseases, where symptoms of senility appear prematurely, or cases of insanity resulting from traumatic injury to the head or from disease. In very few cases would they cover functional mental illness, such as manic-depressive psychosis, schizophrenia, or severe obsessional neuroses, because few competent psychiatrists would care to testify that these conditions are incurable. The *Report* comments:

Apparently, one of the chief ways of determining that a condition is incurable is a showing that the patient has not responded to accepted methods of treatment over a period of time. If the assertion is valid that a majority of patients in state hospitals do not receive adequate treatment because of overcrowding and understaffing, it is difficult to see how an accurate statement in regard to incurability can be made on this basis. There is even greater uncertainty if the criterion is the length of confinement rather than incurability.

It also points out that several of the statutes fail to require that the condition of incurability be established by experts in mental illness, which failure could raise a question in court concerning the reliability of the prognosis given.[4]

Connecticut is unique in specifying that the testimony of incurability be given by two competent psychiatrists who must also be diplomates of the specialty board that governs psychiatry, The American Board of Psychiatry and Neurology.[5] This provision is strange because there is no demonstrated relationship between psychiatric competency and board certification; many competent psychiatrists avoid the Board either because it is open only to members of the American Medical Association or because it requires expert knowledge not only in psychiatry but also in neurology (and thus is the only medical specialty board that demands proficiency in not only the specialty of the examinee but also another discipline). Since most psychiatrists are not diplomates of the Board, and since many of its diplomates represent the nondynamic "old-fashioned" neuropsychiatrists, who are often prognostically pessimistic, the statute, designed probably to give more protection to the hospitalized spouse, has the effect of possibly giving less.

The states that permit a divorce from a hospitalized patient considered incurably ill in most cases require the well spouse to continue to be financially responsible for the sick spouse, and more than half of them specifically provide that this financial responsibility remains the same as though the divorce had not occurred.[6] A provision in the California law, which went so far as to require the plaintiff to prove ownership of property sufficient to support the mentally ill spouse for life, was declared unconstitutional, in 1951, on the ground that this had the effect of "denying divorce to the poor and making it available to the wealthy."[7]

In any event, the psychiatric revolution that commenced with the introduction of thorazine and other tranquilizers has largely nullified the effect of the laws designed to help secure divorces for the well spouses of psychiatric patients. "Incurability" must be certified, and during a time when many patients formerly considered incurable are making satisfactory adjustments to life outside the hospital, it is difficult for many psychiatrists to make such a pessimistic prediction. In "The Need for Prognostic Optimism in Schizophrenic Illnesses," Stephens and Astrup report that two groups of schizophrenic patients were compared, one with a presumably good and one with a presumably poor prognosis. Even in the poor prognosis group, 30% of the patients either required no further hospitalization or were hospitalized for less than one year during the ten years (on an average) follow-up after initial discharge.[8] They cite Holmboe and Astrup, who have reported that they cannot distinguish sharply between poor prognosis cases and atypical schizophrenia with a good prognosis,[9] and they quote a letter written by a patient whose prognosis was considered poor and whose physician predicted chronic hospital care:

I have been working in the post office for several years now and enjoy my work. I get an additional lift in realizing that one branch of the government finds me able to perform my duties even if another considers me permanently disabled. I believe findings such as permanently disabled and incurably insane should have no place in the medical vocabulary. As you know, both these findings have been applied in my case and I have undergone serious hardships because of this.[10]

Since incurability is so hard to determine, a divorce usually cannot be secured from a psychiatrically ill spouse, particularly if the spouse actively opposes the divorce. The effect of this bar to divorce is obvious. When a husband or wife has been in a psychiatric hospital for a long period and no divorce is obtainable, the other partner has frequently entered into a bigamous arrangement or found a partner for adultery, had illegitimate children, and in other ways complicated his or her life for lack of a legal answer in this situation. F. Scott Fitzgerald was one of the notorious partners in such an alliance. When he could not get a divorce from his wife Zelda, hospitalized for schizophrenia, he lived with Sheilah Graham, the Hollywood columnist, for several years, until his death. She has written, in Beloved Infidel, of their life together and the emotional hardships caused by their inability to be married. "I had fallen in love with a man I could not marry. He was married to a woman he could not divorce." When she understood this situation, she became depressed and began to brood.

I was held in a strange spell, a coma, an almost physical paralysis. I was punishing him for not being able to marry me. Yet there was nothing he could do about it. Nor I. I could leave him—but it was impossible for me to imagine life without him. There was nothing to protest; there was nothing to be done; this was the normal injustice of life.[11]

The difficulties that a well spouse has in securing a divorce from a mentally ill spouse are based on the court's desire to protect the helpless. Even if the situation is reversed, if a mentally ill person wants a divorce from a sane person and has such grounds as adultery, desertion or cruelty, only two states allow this action to be brought. In this case, it appears that the court does not seem to want to help the helpless. Even here, however, the philosophy behind state policy seems to be to protect the rights of the psychotic or the hospitalized patient, for, as the American Bar Foundation *Report* points out, "mentally ill persons not infrequently see things in an entirely different light when, if ever, they recover and may not wish to have a divorce after their recovery."[12]

Another category of divorce actions is based on the plea, not that one partner to the marriage has become mentally ill after the marriage, but rather that a mental illness that was not disclosed preexisted, and so the marriage contract was the result of a fraudulent failure to disclose information that should have been disclosed. Courts seem to agree in these cases that a present severe illness—such as the fact that a patient is on leave from a psychiatric hospital—should be disclosed to a prospective spouse and failure to disclose would be grounds for annulment or divorce. On the other hand, past mental illness or past hospitalization would only have to be disclosed in answer to a direct question; the former patient is not at liberty to lie about his past, but he need not volunteer information that is detrimental to his own best interests. Here, as in other matters concerning the law of contracts, the principle of *caveat emptor*, "let the buyer beware," operates.

CHAPTER 8

On the Subject of Wills

COURTS have always been more willing to uphold wills than contracts; the standards of competency to execute a valid will are not
so stringent as those to enter into a binding contract. The main reason
is that in a contract case the claim of incompetency is a defense; the
mentally disabled person is usually the defendant and the plaintiff is
seeking to have him go through with his part of the contract. The
court will allow the contract to stand if it is not disadvantageous to the
patient and if it is shown that his mental illness was not so severe that
it prevented him from understanding the terms of the contract. But
the court—in its capacity as defender of the helpless—will be ready to
strike down the contract if it is not in the best interest of the patient.
In short, releasing the patient from the obligations of a contract that he
has entered into is the way the court helps the helpless.

The party to a contract, unless he is far deteriorated, can assist
his lawyer and help in the defense of a suit. In the case of a will, the
helplessness is more severe. The testator, who had certain wishes about
the disposition of his property that he set forth in a will, so that this
could be accomplished after his death, is now gone; the case could
never have come to court while he was alive. The testator is dead and
now an attempt is being made to break his will, to circumvent the
execution of his express wishes. Allegations are being made about him
—he was senile or delusional or subject to undue influence. Since he
is not there to answer questions and cannot protect himself, the courts
will be anxious to lean over backwards in his favor to put his wishes
into effect. The executor of the will, or the person who is offering the
will for probate, is said to have the burden of proving the testator had
testamentary capacity, but once minimal evidence of the testator's
capacity has been presented, those trying to break the will have the
real task of proving to a doubting court that capacity was lacking.
"The right to dispose of property by will is one which the law is slow
to deny on the ground of lack of testamentary capacity; if such capacity
exists, the court will not undertake to measure its degree."[1]

English common law has recognized documents much like our wills
since the year 1200 or earlier, but these documents were valid only for

the disposition of personal property; real property could not be so bequeathed. In order to clear up many confusions, the English Parliament in 1837 passed the *Statute of Wills*, which gave a statutory basis to the right to make a will and put personal property and real property on the same basis as far as wills were concerned. The first Wills Act granted the right to make a will to everybody without qualifications as to age or sanity. Later, in 1839, the Act was amended to exclude minors, idiots, and "any person de non sane memory." In most United States jurisdictions, laws governing wills are derived from these English laws. The phrase "non sane memory" has been dropped in most statutes and the requirement is usually that the testator must have a "sound mind and memory."

But the standards of soundness of mind and memory are not the same for testamentary capacity as they are for contractual ability or other legal functions. The courts are willing to rule that people who have been adjudicated insane and people who are undeniably psychotic are "of sound mind and memory" so far as will-making ability goes, although they might not be willing to find the same people legally competent to perform any other function. In two jurisdictions—Maryland and the District of Columbia—it is required that testators be capable of making a valid deed or contract, so in these jurisdictions alone persons under guardianship are precluded from making a will.[2]

To have sound mind and memory, for the purposes of will-making, only three criteria need be met:

The testator must be shown to have had that "strength and clearness of mind and memory sufficient to know in general without prompting" *1.* the nature of the act that he is about to perform (he must understand that the document he is signing is a will and he must have a realization of the fact that he is consciously signing it as well as some understanding of the significance of wills); *2.* the nature and extent of the property of which he is about to dispose (he must understand what he is willing away); and *3.* the names and identity of the persons who are the proper objects of his bounty and his relation toward them (he must have sufficient mentation to know, for example, that he has a living wife and children, if he does).[3]

If the testator understands that he is engaging in a devise of his property, knows the nature and extent of his property and can identify the natural objects of his bounty, even though he may be under guardianship or committed to a mental hospital or senile, he can make a valid will.

Who are the natural objects of a testator's bounty? First and foremost, husband and wife, and after that children and parents. Then come less close relatives—brothers and sisters, uncles and aunts, cousins. The natural objects of his bounty must be known to the testator—he cannot think a child who is dead is alive or a child who is alive is dead, and he cannot operate under the hypothesis that his wife is trying to poison him if no evidence for this exists—but he does not have to favor them in his will. If he has enough mental capacity to know who are the important people in his life, he is free to disinherit them. "The fact that a person dislikes his relatives, with or without reason, is not necessarily proof of . . . unsoundness."[4] The practice of leaving one dollar to relatives prevents them from claiming that the testator was so incompetent that he had forgotten that they existed. The concept of knowing the "natural objects of one's bounty" has been loosely defined by courts on various occasions as knowing "friends or relatives or others in whom he feels an especial interest," or recognizing "the claims of others on him for his favorable consideration," or realizing the "deserts and relations to him of those whom he includes in, or excludes from, his will."[5]

Page on Wills gives a slightly amplified version of the criteria for "sound mind":[6]

The use of the term "sound mind" in terms of testamentary capacity does not cause confusion even though the term is not defined by the statutes because a fairly uniform definition of the term has been established by case law. To be of sound mind for the purpose of making a will the testator must be able to:

1. know, without prompting, the nature and extent of the property of which he is about to dispose;
2. know the nature of the act he is about to perform;
3. know the names and identity of the persons who are to be the objects of his bounty;
4. know his relation toward them;
5. have sufficient mind and memory to understand all of these facts;
6. appreciate the relations of these factors to one another;
7. recollect the decision which he has formed.

Courts have said that to void a will, an insane delusion must affect or enter into the execution of the will. The testator can have been psychotic, he can have had delusions of grandiosity or of persecution, but if the aberrations do not appear to have influenced the form of the will or its contents, the court will overlook the psychosis. A Michigan court has said that a man may believe that he is the supreme ruler of the universe, and yet that delusion may not affect the will.[7]

Thus, if a testator states in his will that one son has been kind to him and he is therefore leaving him all of his estate except for one dollar, which is being left to another son who has been unkind, the will would not thereby be invalid. If the disinherited son tries to contest the will by showing that his father had insane delusions concerning being followed, persecuted or the subject of a Communist plot, the will would still not necessarily be invalid. But if the disinherited son could show that his father because of an insane delusion thought his son was conspiring to harm him, then the will would be invalid.

The law tries hard to distinguish between a mistake that is the result of external influence, weighed, however imperfectly, by the reason, and a delusion, which has no basis in external reality. The court has held in one case that the testator's mistaken belief that he was not the father of two children of his divorced wife born during their marriage was not an insane delusion, so as to preclude the probate of a will making no provision for such children if there was any rational basis at all for such a belief.[8] In a somewhat similar will, the court has held that an insane delusion that testator's children were not his own, when there was conclusive evidence of his paternity, voided a will disinheriting the children.[9] Finally, a court has held valid a will written by a testator who had a delusion that his son was trying to kill him but nevertheless left his whole estate to that same son. The court reasoned that here the delusion did not affect the form or content of the will.[10]

The feeling that an insane delusion in itself does not necessarily invalidate a will has strengthened during the last hundred years. At English common law, an insane delusion indicated an unsound mind, and in the early 1800's the doctrine was set down that those of unsound mind could not write valid wills. Isaac Ray—the foremost name in the history of American forensic psychiatry and one of the 13 founders of the Association of Medical Superintendents of American Institutions, which has developed into the American Psychiatric Association—in 1838 published his *Treatise on the Medical Jurisprudence of Insanity*.[11] Ray's view was that "insanity is a disease and, as is the case with all other diseases, the fact of its existence is never established by a single diagnostic symptom, but by the whole body of symptoms, no particular one of which is present in every case." This view of Ray's has been used to uphold two entirely different propositions. In wills cases, it has been used to overthrow the old idea that an insane delusion held by the testator proves the existence of unsoundness of mind (and thus even a delusional testator can be held to be sufficiently well to write a valid will). In criminal cases, it has been used to combat the *M'Naghten Rule* (or rather an overly simplified version of the rule), which holds that if one can distinguish right from wrong he cannot plead insanity as a defense (and thus even a somewhat rational defendant can still be held to be sufficiently unwell to plead insanity as a defense).

Ray's book had been read by New Hampshire's Judge Charles Doe, before writing the dissenting opinion in a wills case of 1866. (Later Ray and Doe entered into an exchange of views that has become noted as the "Doe-Ray Correspondence."[12]) Isaac Ray's thought can be traced through the dissenting opinion of the 1866 wills case to the majority opinion of cases concerning criminal responsibility in New Hampshire from a few years later to the present; now it has become the prevailing opinion in all jurisdictions in wills cases and even in a very few jurisdictions in cases of criminal responsibility. (See Chapter 9, "Criminal Responsibility.")

In his dissent in *Boardman* vs *Woodman*,[13] Judge Doe pointed out that at common law the free operation of a sound mind is the essence of contract and crime, that contracts and crimes do not consist of mere acts or words (but have to be considered in context of their intent), and that they cannot be produced by mental disease. A product of infantile immaturity, according to common law, or of disease of the mind is not a contract, a crime, or a will.

In this case, it had been shown that the testatrix had an insane delusion, and the court ruled on that basis that the will was not valid. Said Judge Doe, dissenting:

> The question whether Miss Blydenburgh had a mental disease was a question of fact for the jury, and not a question of law for the court. Whether delusion is a symptom, or a test, of any mental disease, was also a question of fact, and the instructions given to the jury were erroneous in assuming it to be a question of law. . . . If a jury were instructed that certain manifestations were symptoms or tests of consumption, cholera, congestion, or poison, a verdict rendered in accordance with such instructions would be set aside, not because they were not correct, but because the question of their correctness was one of fact to be determined by the jury upon evidence. Experts may testify to the indications of mental disease, as they could not if such indications were matters of law. . . . Delusion, as a test, seems not to have been heard of in the law before the year 1800, and was not a part of the common law of England when that common law was adopted in our constitution.
>
> The misunderstanding which prevails on this subject, arises from the fact that medical errors of former days gained the sanction, and the name, of law, by being published in law books of high authority. . . .
>
> Insane delusion cannot be adopted as a definition of insanity, on the ground of convenience.[14]

Some authorities have said that if an old and somewhat senile person is making a will, it would be a good idea to have a psychiatric examination done at that time, so that the psychiatrist or his report would be available in the event that there is a court case when the will is filed for probate. It has also been suggested that the psychiatrist might be one of the witnesses to the will.[15] In actual practice, when wills are made out, it is rarely anticipated that court battles will ensue, and if a psychiatrist is a witness there may be an implication that the will-making ability of the testator is borderline, thus casting some doubt on the validity of the will.

In one situation, the courts will not lean over backwards to put the testator's intentions into effect, but will go, often, to the opposite extreme. This is when the testator leaves money to a nurse or a doctor, a minister or a lawyer, or even a close friend, who has been attentive during the final illness, but who is not so close to the testator as other natural objects of bounty. If a man leaves his widow a small portion of his estate but leaves his nurse a large portion, the court will usually rule that this was "undue influence" and the will will therefore be stricken. Mental state enters into this type of attack on a will, because if it can be shown that the testator was very sick, disturbed, dependent on drugs, or had organic brain pathology, to demonstrate suggestibility and probability of "undue influence" is much easier.

When a will is ruled invalid because the testator was of unsound mind, an earlier will written when he was of sound mind, if not destroyed, takes effect. The act of writing a will shows an intent to revoke all previous wills, but if the testator does not have the mental capacity to write a valid will, he also does not have the capacity to revoke the previous will. If no extant will governs the disposition of the property, state laws that govern intestacy will control the distribution of the estate, with various relatives inheriting according to the rules of intestate distribution.

But testacy is preferred to intestacy. The courts will try to find that the author of the will was of sound enough mind to write a valid will. Of all the situations where courts rule on soundness of mind, here standards are most liberal. This is the commonest situation where a person can be insane and still be competent, but to achieve this favored status he must no longer be alive.

CHAPTER 9

Criminal Responsibility

CONTRACTS, WILLS—AND CRIME

A THEME that runs through the law of contracts, wills, and criminal responsibility is the common law doctrine that the intention of the contractor, testator, or perpetrator of an alleged crime is essential to the execution of the contract, will, or crime. As Judge Doe has written:

> The general theory of the common law is, that the free operation of a sound mind is the essence of contract and crime, that contract and crimes do not consist of mere acts or words, and cannot be produced by mental disease. A product of . . . disease of the mind, is not a contract, a crime, or a will.[1]

This principle commands general agreement as regards contracts and wills, but it gives rise to controversy in the area of criminal law. It is true that crimes do not consist of mere acts and that an intention must accompany the act, but it is only true in some jurisdictions that the intention that is an essential element of a crime cannot be formed in the mind of a mentally ill person.

INSANITY AS A DEFENSE

As far back as 1326, in the time of Edward II, the rule had been set forth that madness, later termed insanity, would relieve an accused criminal of the responsibility for his action.[2] (Insanity is not a medical or a psychiatric term; it is entirely a legal term. A patient may be psychotic, but the law acts upon the assumption that he is not insane until there is a judicial determination that he is insane. A hospital inmate who is not psychotic but who has been judicially declared insane *is* insane so long as there has been no legal proceeding that changes this determination. An analogy exists in criminal law. A man may commit a murder but may be declared not guilty by the court. Even though he later admits the crime, he remains not guilty, and because of the laws concerning double jeopardy, cannot be tried again, and so still remains not guilty.)

The defense of insanity was well, but not consistently, recognized in English criminal law. During centuries when small children were sent to the gallows for picking pockets and witches were burned, pity for malefactors was not conspicuous, and whether the accused was exonerated on this ground might depend on his station of life and the mood of the court. During Queen Victoria's reign, this defense was successfully pleaded more frequently, and it secured the acquittal of Edward Oxford who, in 1840, made an attempt on the life of the Queen and Prince Albert. Victoria's alarm mounted when, in 1843, the defense also won an acquittal for Daniel M'Naghten (often spelled McNaughton, McNaghten, M'Naughton, M'Naughten, with other variants). This Scotsman from Glasgow had shot and killed Sir Robert Peel's secretary, who was riding in Sir Robert's carriage, under the mistaken impression that the secretary was Sir Robert and impelled by the belief that Peel's Corn Laws had been passed specifically to cause him financial ruin.

A Note in the *New England Journal of Medicine* describes interesting parallels between M'Naghten, James Hadfield, who a generation earlier had been held not guilty by reason of insanity for an attempt on the life of George III, and Lee Harvey Oswald, who assassinated President Kennedy. This Note points out that evidence on Oswald's mental instability, which, had he lived to stand trial, undoubtedly would have been the basis of his defense, might have made new law on the "still very unsettled medicolegal question: the criminal responsibility of mentally ill persons."

The most important cases in English Common Law on criminal responsibility have involved assassination attempts. The first was the trial of James Hadfield, in 1800, for an attempt on the life of George III. There were many parallels in this case to the actions of Lee Harvey Oswald. Both were former servicemen. In each case, there was a connection with another public figure who was physically at the side of the head of state. For Oswald, it was Texas Governor John Connally, who had been Secretary of the Navy and had refused an Oswald request. For Hadfield, it was the Duke of York, under whom he had served. Both Oswald and Hadfield made their attacks by gunfire at public occasions, and both abandoned their weapons at the scene of the crime.

Hadfield had received severe head and brain injuries in battle and was alleged to have suffered psychotic delusions ever since that time. His defense attorney was Thomas Erskine, the foremost barrister in England. . . . The plea of not guilty due to insanity was made by Erskine and won. The law at the time was based upon an earlier assassination attempt upon a high public figure, Lord Ornslow, in 1724. In *Arnold's Case*, the court had held that to establish insanity as a defense, the defendant had to be totally deprived of his reason so that he did not know what he was doing, any more than an infant or a wild beast would have known. Erskine and the Crown Prosecutor in *Hadfield's Case* both spoke of this "wild-beast" test. The *Hadfield* decision is notable in adding the significance of *insane delusions* as a basis for a finding of insanity.

The next great trial of an assassination involved the only successful attempt on the life of an English Prime Minister, Spencer Percival, in 1812. He was shot by a man named Bellingham, who was very quickly brought to trial, found guilty and hanged within a week of the crime. Bellingham had pleaded not guilty by reason of insanity. Lord Mansfield, the judge at his trial, asserted that to have such a defense, the prisoner must be incapable of distinguishing right from wrong. The fact that Bellingham considered his act one of justifiable revenge against the Government's alleged injustice to him, said the judge, was no defense.

The next case was an attempt on the life of Queen Victoria and Prince Albert in 1840. The assailant, Edward Oxford, was found not guilty because of insanity on extensive evidence of insanity in his family and on evidence that he had delusions about being a member of a secret society. *Hadfield's Case* was used as precedent for the finding.

The last great case, the most important in all Common Law on the subject, was the trial of Daniel M'Naughten in 1843. . . . There are again, as in Hadfield, some strange parallels between Oswald and Daniel M'Naughten. Both were political fanatics. Oswald ran off to Russia but returned to commit his crime against his own country. M'Naughten left his native Scotland in fear of imagined persecution by Jesuit priests. He went to France but returned to England, where he believed he was pursued by spies. He believed that the Tories and the Prime Minister were after him because he had voted against them in the last election.[3]

The Queen, interested in upholding law and order, was shocked when M'Naghten was declared not guilty by reason of insanity (in spite of the fact that he had not gone free but had been committed to an insane asylum) and feared that this decision would lead to an open season on her ministers. Mr. Cockburn, in successfully defending M'Naghten, had stated: "I trust that I have satisfied you that the disease of partial insanity can exist, that it can lead to a partial or total aberration of the moral senses and affections, which may render the wretched patient incapable of resisting the delusion." This did not sit well with the Queen or the House of Lords. It approached the defense of irresistible impulse, which has never been regarded in too kind a light in English law. The Victorian point of view was that the fact that one believes he is persecuted by Tories does not justify murder. The House of Lords, after debating the status of the insanity defense, took the unusual step of asking the chief justices of England, the fifteen "Law Lords," to give their individual answers to five questions concerning this defense. From their answers, a composite rule was formulated, now famous as the Rule (or Rules) in *M'Naghten's Case*.

M'NAGHTEN'S RULE

The rule states that insanity in itself is not a defense, and that the accused must be more than merely insane to receive a verdict of not guilty by reason of insanity. He must be "laboring under such a defective reason, from disease of the mind, as not to know the nature and quality of the act he was doing, or if he did know it, that he did not know he was doing what was wrong." This test has been called the "right and wrong" test, and until 1957 it was the sole test in England. It still remains the chief test in England—except in some homicide cases where the principle of diminished responsibility applies—and it is the sole test in most jurisdictions of the United States.

The *M'Naghten* rule holds that a delusion excuses the commission of the crime provided that the situation assumed by the delusion would excuse if the delusion were in fact true, but that the delusion is not an excuse provided the situation assumed by the delusion would not excuse if it were a fact. For example, a patient with paranoid schizophrenia believes that he is the object of a plot. Even if his insane delusion were true, he would not be justified in killing a policeman whom he thought a part of the plot. But if he insanely believed the policeman was armed and had drawn his gun to shoot, he could justifiably shoot the policeman in self-defense, since this would be a valid action for him to take if the delusion were in fact true.

Whitlock has pointed out that before the *M'Naghten* rule, irresistible impulse had sometimes been recognized by English courts as a ground for a plea of not guilty by reason of insanity, but that after the promulgation of the rule, in spite of the fact that the rule has never had statutory backing, the doctrine of irresistible impulse disappeared from English law for more than one hundred years, reappearing—but only applying to murder and not to other crimes—in the Homicide Act of 1957.[4]

As early as 1869, the *M'Naghten* rule was attacked by the Supreme Court of New Hampshire. The rule had been described as "exquisite inhumanity," because under it defendants who are unquestionably mentally ill are judged by the same standards that apply to other defendants if their irrationality does not interfere with their comprehension of their offense and their concept of accepted standards of right and wrong.

The *M'Naghten* rule has been criticized on other grounds. It has never been clear whether the right or wrong the Law Lords used in their test was *legal* or *moral* right or wrong. Sir James Stephen, famous English legal commentator, pointed out this ambiguity in a book published in 1883. His example was a hypothetical case: A kills B with knowledge of his act and its illegality, but under an insane delusion that the murder of B was directed by God and would result in the salvation of the human race. If the word "wrong" means illegal, A's act is a crime. If the word "wrong" means immoral, A would not be criminally responsible for his act.[5]

Judge Cardozo, serving in New York in 1915, wrote the decision in a case involving a man who had murdered a prostitute because he felt he was commanded to do so by Divine will, "as a sacrifice and atonement." In this case,[6] which has since been the law of New York, the court concluded that the "wrong" of the *M'Naghten* rule ought not to be and was not meant to be limited to legal wrong. (The defendant, appealing his conviction, said that his real offense had not been murder but manslaughter and that he had confessed to the greater crime and then feigned insanity in order to protect abortion ring confederates.) Judge Cardozo ruled that the lower court had erred in finding him guilty because it should have been dealing with the concept of moral wrong, not legal wrong—and it is not morally wrong to murder if voices say this is a religious necessity. (But, since in his appeal the defendant had admitted feigning insanity, he did not set aside the conviction.) Courts in Tennessee and Texas have taken the opposite view; since in Texas legal wrong is the criterion in the "right or wrong" test, Jack Ruby's defense for the killing of Oswald could not take advantage of the argument that he knew his act was legally wrong but felt it was morally justified. The Court of Criminal Appeals of England also considers the Rule to refer only to legal wrong.

Other arguments against the *M'Naghten* rule are:

The defense of insanity is available primarily to patients suffering from hallucinations and delusions. It is not available to other patients who seem equally sick to a psychiatrist. A drug addict, for example, might "know" that it is legally and morally wrong to steal medicine for his "fix" or to obtain the "fix," but the knowledge may not be helpful to him. Zilboorg has expressed this distinction: "This fundamental difference between verbal or purely intellectual knowledge and the mysterious other kind of knowledge is familiar to every clinical psychiatrist; it is the difference between knowledge divorced from affect and knowledge so fused with affect that it becomes a human reality."[7]

Also, the decision whether the defendant can differentiate between right and wrong must be given in unequivocal fashion by the testifying psychiatrist, even though, as we have said, modern psychiatry prefers to be relativistic rather than absolutist. If a starving man steals food, it is wrong from the point of view of the man whose food was stolen but not so clearly wrong from the point of view of the hungry man. Psychiatrists are therefore in every case applying their concept of right or wrong to the acts of the accused, in spite of the fact that psychiatrists pride themselves on not being moralists, theologians, or legalists. To quote Zilboorg again: "To force a psychiatrist to talk in terms of the ability to distinguish between right and wrong and of legal responsibility is . . . to force him to violate the Hippocratic Oath, even to violate the oath he takes as a witness to tell the truth and nothing but the truth."[8] Chief Judge Biggs of the United States Court of Appeals for the Third Circuit, in a dissenting opinion has said: "The law, when it requires the psychiatrist to state whether in his opinion the accused is capable of knowing right from wrong, compels the psychiatrist to test guilt or innocence by a concept which has almost no

recognizable reality."[9]   The American Bar Foundation *Report* points out:
"Since the psychiatrist cannot accurately determine the defendant's capacity
to distinguish right from wrong on the basis of his medical expertise, his testimony on this issue is largely conjecture or a reflection of his own personal judg-
ments of whether or not the defendant should be held responsible."[10]

NEW HAMPSHIRE DOCTRINE

In the last century, there was one exception to the universal adop-
tion of the *M'Naghten* rule in all US jurisdictions.   New Hampshire
did not subscribe to it after 1869; it was influenced by the ideas of
Isaac Ray and its own Judge Doe to say that if the criminal action
was the "offspring or product of mental disease," then the accused can
plead not guilty by reason of insanity.

The *New Hampshire* doctrine has always been considered more
liberal than the rule in *M'Naghten's* case because it widened the application of the insanity defense and, even more important procedurally,
it opened the door to testimony and cross-examination relating to the
whole subject of the defendant's mental condition instead of confining
it to the narrow question of the ability to distinguish between right
and wrong.

IRRESISTIBLE IMPULSE

Starting with Alabama in 1886, fifteen states plus all Federal jurisdictions and military courts have added something to the *M'Naghten*
doctrine.   This is the old doctrine of irresistible impulse, which had
some status in English law before it was swept away by the *M'Naghten*
rule.

This test applies to a defendant who may know the nature and
quality of his act and may be aware that it is wrong, but who, nevertheless, may be irresistibly driven to commit a criminal act by an over-
powering impulse resulting from a mental condition.

There has been some confusion surrounding the use of the term
"irresistible impulse."   The so-called irresistible impulse should not be
confused with the "unresisted impulse."   Where reason is temporarily
blinded by anger, jealousy, or other overriding passions not the result
of a mental condition, the irresistible impulse test as stated above does
not apply.   In such instances there is disagreement about the existence
of criminal responsibility.[11]

But even if "irresistible impulse" is differentiated from "unresisted
impulse," questions remain.   Are some impulses resistible, others irresistible, and can these be differentiated from each other?   Can psychiatry help in making this kind of determination?   Philosophical
questions, such as the existence of freedom of will or of psychic deter-

minism, which are involved in any consideration of rules of criminal responsibility, are raised once again. While psychiatrists and philosophers may find themselves at a loss in deciding when an impulse takes over and becomes irresistible, judges may find that the application of this concept gives them additional scope in trying to relieve a defendant from the usual consequences of his offense when he arouses the sympathy of the court.

THE DURHAM RULE

Acting on the belief that the New Hampshire test of insanity was superior to the *M'Naghten* rule, the United States Court of Appeals for the District of Columbia in 1954 promulgated the now famous *Durham* rule,[12] which abrogates the right or wrong formula and substitutes the rule that a defendant must be held not guilty if the jury finds that his act was the product of mental disease or defect. This enables the testifying psychiatrist to present to the jury the whole history of the patient and his entire psychiatric background.

At first hailed as a great advance, the *Durham* decision has now become the subject of much controversy, and it has been adopted in only one other jurisdiction.[13] Lawyers point out that although the *M'Naghten* rule looks narrow, enlightened judges usually have allowed fairly complete psychiatric testimony[14]; that by enlarging the area of testimony to be considered by the jury, the *Durham* rule gives a group of laymen additional duties in passing judgment on extremely complex medical matters; and that, since law is based on precedent, this new standard has had an unsettling effect on the whole field of criminal law. If it were widely adopted, all the thousands of cases in which the *M'Naghten* rule has been clarified and sharpened would be without value as precedent.

Some critics of the *Durham* rule believe that it would turn most or all criminal cases over to the hands of the psychiatrist rather than the penologist, for all crime can be viewed as the product of mental disease. The shortage of psychiatrists has been given as a reason for attacking *Durham* on the grounds of impracticability (and this argument in turn has been demolished on the ground that criminal standards should not be determined by the availability of psychiatric personnel).[15]

The most profound criticism of *Durham*, however, is that it evolved as a reaction not to the *M'Naghten* tests but to a misunderstanding about them. The *M'Naghten* rule was designed not to define insanity but only to mark out from the larger group of defendants with symptoms of mental illness a smaller group so irrational that they should be relieved of criminal responsibility. If the accused fails to meet

M'Naghten's criteria, the court is not saying that he is mentally well; it is saying that some people in our society can possibly be insane and still be sentenced to jail—or even to the gallows or the electric chair— if there is reason to think that a guilty intention was involved in the criminal act. The rule is a formula for differentiating those insane criminals who are irresponsible and therefore permitted to plead an unusual defense from all other defendants, sane or insane.

If *Durham* says that in the light of the impact of psychiatric knowledge on contemporary morality this formula no longer represents social morals, and that today seriously disturbed offenders should not suffer the stigma of criminal conviction but be hospitalized instead of jailed, then it seeks to revolutionize concepts of criminal responsibility rather than modernize a definition to accommodate a wider scope of psychiatric testimony. Under this view, most prisoners—being character neurotics and psychopathic personalities—should be reclassified as patients. Obviously, such does not reflect the moral view of the Law Lords: by setting higher standards, they were not oblivious to the facts of mental life, but they were saying that insanity per se is no excuse for committing a crime.

AMERICAN LAW INSTITUTE TEST

The American Law Institute *Model Penal Code*, Tentative Draft No. 4, explicitly rejects the *Durham* rule,[16] calling attention to the words requiring the unlawful act to be "the product of mental disease or defect." The difficulty with this formulation inheres in the ambiguity of "product." Does this mean that a defendant is not responsible unless had he not suffered from disease or defect he still would have committed the same crime? Then the formulation is too broad because "an answer that he would have done so can be given very rarely. . . . If interpreted to call for a standard of causality less relaxed than but-for-cause, there are but two alternatives to be considered: 1. a mode of causality involving total incapacity or 2. a mode of causality which involves substantial incapacity. . . . But if either of these causal concepts is intended, the formulation ought to set it forth."

The *Model Penal Code* presents a test that provides:

1. A person is not responsible for criminal conduct if at the time of such conduct as a result of mental disease or defect he lacks substantial capacity either to appreciate the criminality of his conduct or to conform his conduct to the requirements of law.

2. The terms "mental disease or defect" do not include an abnormality manifested only by repeated criminal or otherwise antisocial conduct.[17]

Vermont in 1959 and Illinois in 1961 adopted the American Law Institute test, and Maine in 1961 adopted the *Durham* rule. New York in 1965 also abandoned *M'Naghten* by a statute that replaces the test of "knowing" by the concept of "lack of substantial capacity" to know and appreciate the nature of the act by reason of mental disease or defect; this statute also widens the scope of psychiatric testimony. The definition adopted by Vermont speaks of the defendant's "adequate capacity either to appreciate the criminality of his conduct or to conform his conduct to the requirements of the law." These four states and New Hampshire have abandoned *M'Naghten*; 45 states still adhere either to *M'Naghten* alone or *M'Naghten* plus irresistible impulse.

Three additional Federal jurisdictions have also abandoned *M'Naghten*. The United States Court of Appeals for the Third Circuit, a Federal jurisdiction embracing Pennsylvania, New Jersey, Delaware and the Virgin Islands, promulgated a test using the concept that the mental disease or defect must be such that as a result the defendant lacks substantial capacity to conform his conduct to the requirements of the law.[18] This formulation, by Judge John Biggs, was a response to his feeling that the *Durham* rule represented an improvement on *M'Naghten* but was too broad since perhaps all criminality can be considered a product of mental disease or defect; it is known as the *Currens* test. At Judge Bigg's suggestion, the Virgin Islands also passed a statute liberalizing its rule of criminal responsibility.[19] The Tenth Circuit in 1963, after considering *Durham* and *Currens*, adopted the philosophy of the American Law Institute test: the members of the jury must be instructed that "before they may return a verdict of guilty, they must be convinced beyond a reasonable doubt that at the time the accused committed the unlawful act he was mentally capable of knowing what he was doing, was mentally capable of knowing that it was wrong, and was mentally capable of controlling his conduct."[20]

ABOLISH THE DEFENSE?

All the problems we are considering—the battle of the experts, the extent of the defendant's responsibility, the tests to determine the responsibility—would disappear if the legislatures and the courts should decide to abolish the defense of insanity. In one fell swoop, all discussion of *M'Naghten*, irresistible impulse, the *New Hampshire* rule, *Durham*, the *Model Penal Code*, and *Currens* become irrelevant. Abolition of the insanity plea has been argued by both psychiatrist and lawyer. Dr. John McDonald, psychiatrist, would abolish the insanity plea "in the best interests of society and the rehabilitation of the sick man. . . . When people can get off punishment by pleading insanity, they will plead this more often. It would be unfortunate if we liberalized the rules and turned our mental institutions into penitentiaries."[21] Judge Warren E. Burger of the United States Court of Appeals, District of Columbia, states that "the adversary system with all its clash and partisan contention is simply not attuned to the nuances of psychiatry, and we waste these talents when we try to use them in the pointless quest to resolve the issue of criminal responsibility in that atmosphere."[22]

These experts believe that abolition of the insanity defense and the reservation of the question of insanity for "impartial" pre- or post-trial determination would not deprive defendants of important legal safeguards. Most commentators do not agree.

PURPOSEFUL CONTROVERSY?

This complicated controversy—with its overtones of semantic quibbles and theological and philosophical inquiries into such areas as the concept of "free will"—continues to rage, and possibly to no purpose.

The most striking application of the insanity defense rule is in cases involving capital punishment for murder. In lesser crimes, defendants who could possibly plead insanity are reluctant to do so—even criminals dislike to stigmatize themselves as "crazy"—and if the defense is successfully pleaded, the defendant may pave the way for an indeterminate stay in a psychiatric hospital, which may not seem to him as desirable as a fixed stay in a prison. As the idea of capital punishment fades from the American scene, as it has faded in Britain, some of the difficulties in determining criminal responsibility will disappear with it. In crimes where the death penalty is not involved, the question whether a disturbed individual who has admittedly done an illegal act should go to prison (where he could, hopefully, receive psychiatric treatment) or to a state hospital (where he could, hopefully, receive psychiatric treatment) might often be meaningless because neither of the two alternatives is clearly superior to the other.

It has been said, with good reason, that there are few occasions when an accused man pleads insanity or diminished responsibility unless there is a likelihood that he will receive a capital sentence should he be convicted. The possibility of an indefinite period in Broadmoor Hospital rather than a limited prison sentence is only to be preferred when the alternative is death. No doubt there will be many occasions when it is vital that the state of mind of the defendant should be inquired into to ensure that an insane person receives proper treatment rather than that he should be sent to prison with the possibility of a repetition of a serious offence on discharge. There will, in consequence, always be a place for proper and careful psychiatric examination of certain classes of offenders so that the courts may be guided in coming to a right conclusion about the disposal of the defendant. Yet it could be said that only when the charge is a capital one does the sanity or insanity of the defendant become of such crucial importance as to make it seem as if all that matters is the outcome of a conflict of medical opinion . . .[23]

DIMINISHED RESPONSIBILITY

This English view refers to the concept of diminished responsibility, a principle in the law of Scotland dating back to 1867, under which the court can instruct the jury that it is within its discretion to return a lesser degree than murder—culpable homicide, which does not carry with it the death penalty—if it believes that the prisoner's mental state would be adequate justification for the lesser verdict. Scottish cases in which this verdict have been rendered include murders by epileptics, mental defectives, alcoholics and persons suffering from conditions "bordering on insanity," but not by persons merely intoxicated. This doctrine of diminished responsibility was made a part of the law of England by the Homicide Act of 1957.

DETERMINATION OF SANITY FOR OTHER PURPOSES

The question of the defendant's sanity appears at two other stages of the trial and posttrial procedure, but in these cases the *M'Naghten* rule does not apply, since the relevant test is not of right or wrong but of sufficient mentation to understand what is going on. When a defendant is insane, he is not allowed to stand trial, the theory being that only a sane person can cooperate with his counsel in his own defense. The trial is postponed until the defendant is no longer under an adjudication of insanity. Also, when a convicted defendant is sentenced to die but as the day of execution approaches is found to be insane, he cannot be executed. An early principle of the law was that capital punishment was meant primarily for the edification and instruction of society, and it has long been felt in English law that putting an insane person to death would not advance society or edify the populace.

Sometimes, but very rarely, an admitted murderer falls between two stools and escapes punishment because of the workings of the laws regarding insanity. A kills B in an unmotivated crime. He is held to be not guilty because of insanity. The question that then arises is, Should there now be an adjudication of insanity so that A can be incarcerated not in a prison but in a mental hospital? But the court may rule that although A was insane at the time of the murder—hence his guiltlessness—he has now recovered his sanity. By the time the alienation hearing is held, there is no longer a basis for commitment to a mental hospital. Although public feeling opposes crime without punishment, this sequence of sanity and insanity does occur—but not frequently.

A new complication in the definition of sanity was called to the attention of the American Academy of Forensic Sciences by Dr. Werner Tuteur at a recent meeting.[24] A psychiatrist, Dr. Tuteur said that the question whether psychotics in remission as a result of tranquilizer therapy are to be considered insane or sane introduces a new, challenging complication into forensic psychiatry. "It is by now well known that adequate doses of tranquilizers alleviate paranoid thinking and that this alleviation continues to exist for a considerable length of time after discontinuation of the medication given." He cited two cases.

An Air Force enlisted man was treated for a paranoid schizophrenic reaction with tranquilizers and discharged from the service. He then participated in an armed robbery. During a psychiatric examination, he showed symptoms of dissatisfaction with life and suggestibility but did not express delusional thinking. The psychiatrist saw him as still basically a schizophrenic person, although now this was not clearcut because the delusions had disappeared under the influence of the tranquilizer.

In another case, a man was charged with murder in 1955. He was not able to stand trial because he was declared legally insane, and remained in an Illinois mental hospital until 1964. Hospital reports indicated his paranoid delusions disappeared on tranquilizers. In 1964, he was declared legally sane and then tried for the 1955 crime. The jury found him guilty and asked for the death penalty. "A catastrophe was avoided by the court," said Dr. Tuteur, "which sentenced him to 30 to 50 years in the penitentiary instead."[25]

PURPOSE OF IMPRISONMENT

Some psychiatrists and lawyers have observed that the answer to the problem of criminal responsibility is obscured by the fact that society does not know why it imprisons its criminals. Sometimes the rationale seems to be to deter others, sometimes to treat the criminal and to reeducate him, most often to punish him. It has been suggested, hopefully, that if therapy for the emotionally ill criminal was a main goal of society, the decision between prison or hospital might depend on treatability rather than state of mind. Judge David Bazelon, who wrote the majority opinion in the *Durham* case, has recently suggested that community health centers could treat criminals as an alternative to prison isolation, and that this would also help the community in understanding the criminal.[26]

But criminals are the most difficult patients for a psychiatrist to treat, and most psychiatrists do not want to fill the state posts that would make more psychiatric treatment available for criminals.

Except for a relatively small number of posts the money and prestige which are important in this society tend to lie elsewhere than in our public institutions and projects. The best people can only be attracted by a judicious combination of money, academic or other organizational prestige, and an area in which they can function independently in order to realize goals which they themselves consider significant. It would be completely unrealistic, for example, to expect our most talented . . . to abandon prestigious or lucrative careers in other areas in order to work in institutions dominated by less adequate people than they and hampered by rigid, tradition-bound structures.[27]

FIXING RESPONSIBILITY

Psychiatrists and lawyers must face the question whether any "rule" or "test" will ever definitely fix responsibility, and the related question whether a new test will produce superior justice or better rehabilitative efforts for prisoners than M'Naghten. Two compelling reasons argue against change.

First, unless some extreme position is drawn—for instance, unless all offenders are considered ill, or no offenders are considered ill, or the defense of insanity is abolished—the question of the legal responsibility of the defendant will be at issue, which will in our tradition involve questions concerning his state of mind and extent of control over his own actions. Whether liberal or narrow concepts of mental illness prevail will then depend not entirely on the wording of the "test" or "rule": the emotional climate prevailing in society, the philosophy of the judge, the prejudices of the jury will continue to be more important than the wording of the "test." In a peaceful and prosperous society, the emphasis will probably shift towards rehabilitation and less emphasis on guilt; in a threatened society, the emphasis will shift towards punishment and deterrence. Economic factors, the tensions prevailing in society, the extent of knowledge, the understanding in society of psychiatric concepts, the concepts of what society is trying to accomplish—all these are more important than the wording of a "test." In light of the facts that psychiatric knowledge is presently unsettled, that psychiatric concepts are generally unaccepted, and that the adversary procedure provides important safeguards for the defendant, the final determination of guilt or innocence will probably be made by a jury and not the panel or impartial expert sometimes advocated. But whoever makes the determination is acted on by the forces of the world in which he lives. Any "test" in time is shaped to the mood of that time.

Second, the M'Naghten rules have not always been and need not be narrow. True, "hanging judges" who do not wish to give much weight to psychiatric testimony can restrict it to the narrow question of ability to determine right from wrong, but more permissive judges will give weight to broader psychiatric testimony, including childhood influences, in determining whether the defendant comes under either of *M'Naghten's* tests. If a prisoner is insane, the application of the tests can be consistent with Maudsley's statement in 1874: "Of few insane persons who do violence can it be truly said that they have a full knowledge of the nature and quality of their acts at the time they are doing them."[28]

Working within the framework of present legal concepts, the job remains of setting the line which divides criminal responsibility from innocence by reason of state of mind. The line will undoubtedly be determined in the future, as it has in the past, not by the wording of tests but by the feeling of society, divided in its desire to protect itself and to be humane. Judge Jerome N. Frank has defined the two opposing extremes: "Society must be protected against violence and at the same time avoid punishing sick men whose violence drives them beyond their controls to brutal deeds. A society that punishes the sick is not wholly civilized. A society that does not restrain the dangerous madman lacks common sense."[29]

The issues are defined; it is only the solutions that await determination.

CHAPTER 10

Informed Consent and Disclosure

WHEN we come to the subject of informed consent, our themes become less clear and sometimes almost disappear. This is an aspect of law where the principles of special attention to the helpless, the necessity of assent, and the protection of the rights of individuals are, for good or bad reasons, neglected.

When the patient is not a psychiatric patient, the law tends to follow its normal course and our themes are usually evident. For example, a Canadian appeal court recently awarded damages of $104,131 to a 38-year-old woman paralyzed following spinal anesthesia. The patient had told the surgeon and the anesthetist that she wanted a general anesthetic, but after receiving sedation she was prevailed on to accept a spinal anesthetic. She became permanently paralyzed below the waist. There being no evidence of negligence, the trial was brought on the issue whether the patient had consented to the type of anesthesia used. The ruling of the court was that the doctor may not overrule his patient and submit his patient to risks that the patient is unwilling to accept. Here, the fact that the consent had finally been given only when the patient was not in full control of her faculties, when she was under sedation, led to the decision against the hospital and its chief anesthetist.[1]

CONSENT AND MENTAL ILLNESS

When consent is required from a patient who is mentally ill, even more than from a patient who is merely under sedation, three questions will obviously be raised. One, does a consent to a procedure have to be secured from a mental patient in the same manner that is required from other patients? Two, did the patient fully understand the procedure that he was to undergo and its risks? Three, does a mental patient have the authority to give his own consent or has this function been assumed by someone who is presumably better able to understand the implications of the procedure, perhaps by physicians representing the state itself? These are the same questions that arise when

68

a minor—another category that the law considers less than competent —has to undergo surgery or some other potentially dangerous procedure, except that here the parent or one standing in the place of the parent would be the person, presumably better able to understand, who would give final consent.

Moritz and Stetler, in their *Handbook of Legal Medicine*, give some of the general law as it applies to all patients. A physician who treats or operates on a patient without having authority to do so, expressed (written or oral) or implied, commits an assault and battery for which he may be prosecuted criminally or held civilly liable. The rule is subject to exception in an emergency.

> The consent given must be an informed consent with an understanding of what is to be done and of the risks involved. The procedure involved and its attendant risks should be explained to the patient in understandable, non-technical terms. . . .
> Although the law is not yet precisely defined, the holdings in recent cases involving alleged lack of consent may make the physician a frequent target for professional liability claims whenever a bad result occurs. Since the gist of the action does not involve negligent treatment but negligence in failing to explain the hazards to the patient, the claim of alleged lack of informed consent may develop a new "theory" of liability against physicians. Under the circumstances, the physician must be prepared to prove in court that he explained the risks involved to the patient whenever surgical, therapeutic, or diagnostic procedures involve more than the hazards which the patient might normally expect. The physician's best protection is to inform the patient fully regarding any unusual risks that may be involved and to insist upon a consent in writing in which the patient acknowledges this explanation.[2]

Concerning the mentally disabled, they say:

> If the patient is of unsound mind and is incompetent to understand the nature, purpose, and risks incident to a proposed operation . . . authority must come, from his spouse or legally appointed guardian.[3]

Long in his *The Physician and the Law* gives an equally simple rule concerning married women:

> A married woman of sound mind has the power to consent to a surgical operation. When the wife is mentally incompetent the consent of the guardian should be obtained, and if there is a question of mental competence the consent of the husband should be obtained.[4]

Although in some jurisdictions a minor in his late teens may consent to a simple surgical procedure, the general rule is that "the parent is the only one who can legally give consent . . . and if consent is not given, a surgeon's act in performing the operation amounts to technical assault and battery for which the child may recover."

The law reposes in the parent the care and custody of the minor child, and neither a physician nor those in temporary custody of the child may be permitted to determine those matters touching its welfare.[5] The only exception is in an emergency, wherein the surgeon may take such measures as he considers necessary to preserve life.

The basic law appears simple enough. Yet securing consent from children, the mentally ill, and volunteers in experimental medicine presents complicated problems. These last may be under special pressures to participate—medical students, for example, or prisoners who may receive time off for "volunteering" as subjects—and their consent might be considered to have been secured by "constraint or coercion" in violation of the Nuremberg Code.

The Mentally Disabled and the Law describes some of the problems that follow a decision to subject a mentally ill person to surgery or electroshock and to seek his consent to the proposed procedure. They have arisen often concerning psychosurgery—such as the lobotomy, designed to reduce tension and distress of certain emotional states by amputation of the prefrontal areas of the brain, or the prefrontal leukotomy, in which frontal projection fibers are severed. The candidate for psychosurgery is usually psychotic, and often is considered a chronic case. The patient to receive electric shock therapy may be psychotic or not, and some doctors, whom we have categorized as non-Freudians, give this type of treatment routinely to office patients suffering from obsessions, neurotic anxiety, and other conditions where powers of thinking are usually considered to be relatively unimpaired.

The *Report* notes that "one school of thought maintains that public mental hospitals need not obtain consent for surgery . . ."[6] and quotes Ross:

> The argument is that mentally ill persons are considered wards of the state. The state as *parens patriae* must provide necessary care and treatment. The care and treatment of mental patients is a governmental function, and the basic consideration in the exercise of this function is the patient's welfare, not what the patient or his relatives believe to be in his interests.[7]

The *Report* takes a less extreme position. It notes that some states have administrative regulations requiring consent for brain surgery or lobotomy, and that the major nature of this type of treatment—which is controversial, drastic, and irreversible—possibly raises doubt whether the state acting as a parent can supply consent.

The lobotomy has fallen into disrepute, although before it fell from favor, it has been estimated that more than 30,000 of these operations had been done in the United States. Dr. Walter Freeman, who introduced the technic of the lobotomy to the United States in the

1930's, sees the trend against the lobotomy as reversed and has reported that the operation has been increasingly used since 1963, particularly in the West and Southwest. But other observers see the operation as of dubious validity, still debatable after three decades; a study in the *Canadian Medical Association Journal* of two groups of 183 matched mental patients—one group lobotomized and one group not—showed that five years postoperatively 79 patients in the operated group had been discharged from the hospital compared to 68 in the control group, a statistically insignificant difference.[8]

What is the general policy of mental hospitals regarding the necessity of the consent of their patients for major medical treatment?

Many states consider all mental patients incompetent, and therefore their consent might be considered ineffective by a court. Many patients do not have estates and, consequently, in some states do not have guardians. Others may have become estranged from their families or may be hospitalized in places away from their own communities. Even if the patient is competent, there would be a question of whether he would be likely to withhold his consent when his release from the hospital and his other personal rights are determined primarily by the hospital officials seeking his consent.

A few states have dealt with this problem by statute. Illinois specifically and uniquely provides that consent is not necessary, while Ohio and Oklahoma require that relatives be notified of a major operation except in emergency cases. Ohio includes the personal or family physician of the patient, his spouse, parent, guardian or one of his next of kin. The Ohio statute requires notice rather than consent. . . .[9]

Only six states have statutory provisions concerning the mentally disabled and consent for surgery. In all other states, hospitals depend on general language, which does not specifically cover surgery, to give them power to treat the patient. The approach is a practical one, particularly since many patients remain responsibilities of the state after their families have died or lost interest in them, and many patients are hospitalized in parts of the country far from their original homes, where their families may still reside. But although the approach is practical, there is room for question whether the law is its usual vigilant self.

The American Bar Foundation *Report* notes that there are no statutes or cases dealing with consent for electroshock treatment, and the only available detailed discussion is an advisory opinion of the Pennsylvania Department of Justice. It states that superintendents of state mental hospitals may administer these and other treatments that they consider "necessary and proper for the patients' best welfare, without first obtaining written permission for such treatments from such patients, their friends, relatives, guardians or other persons who may be legally entitled to give such consent on behalf of such patients; while such consent may be desirable in some cases, it is not essential under the laws of this Commonwealth."[10]   In the absence of a legal ruling, states have administratively decided that consent from a legally responsible person (Michigan or New York) is necessary or, at the other end of the spectrum, that no consent is needed (Kentucky). Sometimes individuals not considered mentally incompetent, such as sexual offenders, are in a mental hospital on court order; in many jurisdictions, they can be subjected to surgery, including psychosurgery, or to such procedures as electroshock, without their consent.[11]

One state, Kansas, specifically bars patients in state hospitals from recovering damages after suffering injury from shock treatment if the treatment is given in an accepted manner—unless gross negligence can be shown.   The American Bar Foundation *Report* notes that this statute and the sparse case law on the subject, in which the finding in every case was for the defendant physician or hospital, make it difficult for the patient either to protect himself from injury or to recover damages for negligence or gross negligence, inasmuch as he is often forced to submit to the treatment and is unable to testify about what happened to him while he was unconscious.   In addition, the patient is not extended the privilege of selecting a physician or technician who he believes will observe the necessary precautions.

The law's willingness to hold the attending physician harmless from liability for physical injuries due to electroshock treatment points up the drastic aspect of the therapy and underscores the desirability of a consensual relationship between the patient and the doctor.

Since both electroshock treatment and psychosurgery may have very serious consequences, and since there is some question of their medical usefulness, it behooves lawmakers to consider seriously the enactment of measures designed to protect against improper use of these technics.[12]

CONSENT AND SCIENTIFIC EXPERIMENTATION

A major conflict of medicine, law, and morality has centered in the doctrine of informed consent applicable to all medical patients who are the subjects of scientific experiments.   During recent decades, as efforts have been made to make medicine increasingly scientific and as the principle of controlled experimentation, rather than random clinical observations, has come to the fore in medical research, numberless patients have played unwitting parts in research programs.   The efficacy of a drug or a procedure is no longer merely a matter for the judgment of the individual prescribing physician; it is based increasingly on double-blind studies, matched sample populations, and other technics associated with statistical probability theory, and these involve comparisons of patients receiving and patients not receiving treatment.

A new drug or a new technic raises questions of obligation— medical, legal and ethical—not only to the patient who will be administered the new and untried therapy, but to the patient in the next bed who is being deprived, in the interests of science, of the opportunity for a possibly life-saving treatment. Should a patient be maintained in a hospital on no treatment because he is part of a group chosen to receive placebos rather than active medication? Is there an obligation to tell the patient who is receiving a placebo that the drug he is receiving may or may not be a real drug? If the disclosure is not made, then the patient is receiving no treatment when he believes that he is receiving treatment and when he has given no consent to this lack of therapy. But, on the other hand, if the disclosure is made, it will almost certainly affect the outcome of the experiment, since the fact that a patient knows that the medication he is taking may be a placebo will alter his subjective response to the medication or lack of it.

The subject of the transplant of one of a set of paired organs from a mentally incompetent donor, who may not realize the risk of the operation, to a close relative who requires an organ that has a maximum chance of continuing to function in the new host raises questions. So does the related question of the appropriateness of organ transplant to a child or mentally incompetent recipient. Concerning the value of the recipient to society, the doctor is forced to assume an omnipotent role. A Denver team, consisting of three surgeons who work together on kidney transplants, states that a patient is treated "if it is thought that this can be successfully done, and if there is a reasonable chance that the patient will be able to assume a useful place in society. Children, whose social worth is not yet known, cannot be reasonably excluded. Mental defectives, or those with serious concomitant disease, advanced age, major abnormalities of the lower urinary tract, or serious coexistent infections, would not then be considered. The decisions are, therefore, made on the basis of medical criteria."[13] They add that homotransplantation would not be performed in an unwilling or mentally incompetent recipient.

Turning from the recipient to the donor, Paul Freund, professor at the Harvard Law School, has commented on the "special problem of subjects not possessed of full capacity to consent, in particular the problem of children."[14]

The law here is that parents may consent for the child if the invasion of the child's body is for the child's welfare or benefit. This has become familiar through the kidney-transplant cases, in which the Massachusetts Supreme

Judicial Court was asked to render an advisory opinion. Benefit was found to exist in the psychic welfare of the normal donor brother because, after considerable interrogation of the normal child, it was concluded that he would be suffering under some feeling of inadequacy if he did not make the donation, and so the transplants were judicially approved. But what of unrelated donors, who will become more important as transplants between strangers become more feasible? Shall children be ineligible, since it would be hard to find any benefit to the donor child in the transplant with a stranger and the parent seems legally incapable of giving consent in the absence of benefit to the child? It may be that the result is that children will be ineligible as donors for transplants, unless, perhaps—and here we have some other variables—the risk is relatively slight. Might benefit be found on the monetary side?

Coming to that, what of the giving of payment as it may affect the reality of consent? I would suggest that the amounts paid should not be so large as to constitute undue influence—that is, so large as to obscure an appreciation of the risk and weaken the will to self-preservation. We ought not to be put in the business of buying lives.

Freund also discusses the use in experimental research of students (who are not minors) and that other class subject to coercion and undue influence, prisoners. Regarding students, he commends the system at Harvard Medical School, where the investigators, the administrative board, and the Department of Environmental Health must all give approval for their employment as volunteer subjects. Regarding prisoners, he recommends that there should be no promises of parole or commutation of sentence:

this would be what is called in the law of confessions undue influence or duress through promises of reward, which can be as effective in overbearing the will as threats of harm. Nor should there be a pressure to conform within the prison generated by the pattern of rejecting parole applications of those who do not participate. It should not be made informally a condition of parole that one go along, be a good prisoner and subject himself to medical experimentation.[15]

The same week that Freund's recommendations were published in the *New England Journal of Medicine*, a medical newspaper reported that two pharmaceutical companies have built laboratories on the grounds of the state prison of southern Michigan at Jackson, in order to test drugs more rapidly and to supervise volunteers continuously.[16]

Are the problems of informed consent in experimental medicine unsolvable? A newspaper roundup on the subject[17] has pointed out the strict position of the Nuremberg Code, formulated by the Nazi War Crimes Commission and aimed at preventing a repetition of those atrocities committed in the name of medical science in German concentration camps. This ten-point code has no validity in law, but it has been the basis for subsequent formulations and is considered the standard for the ethics of experimentation. It states that in medical research of this kind, "the voluntary consent of the human subject is absolutely essential."

This means that the person involved should have legal capacity to give consent, be able to exercise free power of choice without the intervention of any element of force, fraud, deceit, duress, overreaching, or other ulterior form of constraint or coercion, and have sufficient knowledge and comprehension of the elements of the subject matter involved as to enable him to make an understanding and enlightened decision. This latter element requires that before the acceptance of an affirmative decision by the experimental subject, there should be made known to him the nature, duration, and purpose of the experiment, and the method and means by which it is to be conducted; all inconveniences and hazards reasonably to be expected; and the effects on his health or person which may possibly come from his participation in the experiment.

The duty and responsibility for ascertaining the quality of the consent rests on each individual who initiates, directs, or engages in the experiment. It is the personal duty and responsibility that may not be delegated to another with impunity.

Physicians queried included Dr. Henry Beecher, Professor of Research in Anaesthesia at Harvard Medical School and Director of the Department of Anaesthesia at Massachusetts General Hospital, and Dr. Walter Modell, Director of Clinical Pharmacology at Cornell University School of Medicine. Dr. Beecher cited the problem of communicating risks to the incompetent, among which he included not only infants and children and the mentally deficient, but also the laymen who do not have the background to enable them to comprehend a complex technical proposal. He also questioned the use of civil prisoners, medical students, and other "captive" groups in whom coercive pressure, however subtle, might be experienced. Dr. Modell, on the other hand, felt "that when society confers the degree of physician on a man it instructs him to experiment on his fellow," and that "when a patient goes to a modern physician for treatment, regardless of whether he consciously consents to it, he is also unconsciously presenting himself for the purpose of experimentation."

Even Dr. Modell's authoritarian view is less extreme than the position of an eminent Italian surgeon who spoke recently at a meeting in New York. Said Dr. Achille Dogliotti, Professor of Surgery at the University of Turin: "The surgeon, because of his lofty mission, should have complete scientific and moral independence, especially in regard to the law." The practice of requiring written consent for surgical procedures "must be considered a mortifying sign of low-grade public morality, in which a man's word of honor has lost its value. In a civilized country, with an enlightened judiciary, it should not be necessary."[18]

Lawyers as well as doctors have come face to face with the problems related to experimental design and the difficulties in using humans as research subjects. Freund gives two examples:

In the end, we may have to accept the fact that some limits do exist to the search for knowledge. The legal profession learned this painfully a few years ago in connection with the so-called jury experiment at the University of Chicago, conducted with the sponsorship of a great foundation, where electronic eavesdropping was practiced in various jury rooms to learn what actually goes on in the confines and confidence of that chamber. This was done with the approval of the judge and of counsel in the case but, of course, in the ignorance of members of the jury themselves. When, somehow, news of this leaked out, there was a tremendous furor in legal and public circles, and the experiment was abandoned.[19]

A juvenile-court judge of rather progressive and scientific mind decided to try an experiment regarding sentencing. There were two institutions available: one an ordinary prison; and the other a minimum-security institution where the offenders would return in the evening after being allowed to go out into the town and work during the day. In sentencing to one or the other place of detention, this judge was not inclined to weight the merits of the individual offenders or appraise the likelihood of their benefiting from one rather than the other form of treatment. What he did was to pair off the offenders coming before him in the best way he could, in point of age, ethnic grouping, intelligent quotient, family background and so on; one of the pair would be sent to one place of correction and the other to the other, and the plan was that at intervals careful observations would be made so that in the future there would be some basis for judging the kind of offender who can be expected to profit or not to profit from one or another type of treatment. Perhaps I should not be disturbed by this, but I am troubled because it seems to be an unprincipled way of taking liberties with the liberty of young offenders—unprincipled, that is, except from the standpoint of experimental design. I would be a little easier in my mind if this experiment were thought to be of benefit to the particular offenders who are being sentenced, rather than to their successors or their children.[20]

Of the various codes that have been devised since the Nuremberg Code to deal with the subject of human experimentation, the best known is that of the World Medical Association. The final draft, known as the *Declaration of Helsinki*, was accepted at the meeting of that group held in Finland in June 1964. Dealing with clinical research combined with professional care (Therapeutic Clinical Research), the Declaration states that the doctor must be free to use a new therapeutic measure if he feels it offers hope of saving life, reestablishing health, or alleviating suffering. It then adds:

If at all possible, consistent with patient psychology, the doctor should obtain the patient's freely given consent after the patient has been given a full explanation. In case of legal incapacity consent should also be procured from the legal guardian; in case of physical incapacity the permission of the legal guardian replaces that of the patient.

Clinical research can be combined with professional care only to the extent that clinical research is justified by its therapeutic value for the patient.

Concerning nontherapeutic clinical research—a more difficult problem, since there is no possibility of improvement of a medical condition of the subject—the *Declaration* emphasizes that it is the duty of the doctor to remain the protector of the life and health of that person on whom the clinical research is being carried out, that the subject must be informed about the nature, the purpose, and the risk of the research, and that the research cannot be undertaken without the free consent of the subject after he has been fully informed. A subject legally incompetent may participate in the research if his legal guardian consents, but although legally incompetent, he must understand fully the risks and be able to assert himself: "The subject of clinical research should be in such a mental, physical, and legal state as to be able to exercise fully his power of choice." The investigator must respect the right of each individual to safeguard his personal integrity, especially if the subject is in a dependent relationship to the investigator.

DISCLOSURE OF SIDE-EFFECTS

Besides getting consent for surgery, procedures, and experiments, physicians have the duty to inform their patients concerning the possible risks and side-effects of prescribed medication. A recent Washington State case concerned a bus driver, who had a nasal condition for which an antihistamine was prescribed. While driving the bus, he fell asleep or blacked out, and the bus left the road. Sued by an injured passenger, he cited the physician's failure to disclose that drowsiness was a possible side-effect of the medication. Although the judgment in the lower court was in favor of the physician, the Washington State Supreme Court reversed it and ordered a new trial, holding that there was sufficient evidence to sustain a jury finding that the physician was negligent, and that this negligence was the proximate cause of the passenger's injuries.[21]

The implications of this decision for psychiatry are enormous. When tranquilizers and other medications are prescribed, ample evidence indicates that they can cause a host of side-effects, many of which might slow reflexes, cause drowsiness, and impair judgment. It is interesting to speculate how many auto accidents and industrial accidents have been caused by medication and whether the prescribing physicians had warned the patients of all possible side-effects. One psychiatrist who recently raised this question countered it with the more optimistic possibility that the patients driving cars or running machines under the influence of tranquilizers possibly represent a better risk drugged than they would nervous. In any case, practicing psychiatrists know that if all the possible side-effects of commonly prescribed tranquilizers were listed for the patient—agranulocytosis, photosensitivity and skin eruptions, Parkinson-like symptoms, corneal opacities: the list continues—the disease might seem often preferable to the cure, and patients would refuse the medication.

CHAPTER 11

Sterilization and Abortion

WHETHER human lives should be brought into being has become a question for psychiatry, although many psychiatrists resent being asked to take responsibility for a decision of this type and magnitude.

Psychiatrists can become involved in three ways, most often when they advise a patient to have or not to have children, or additional children. Here the psychiatrist is being directive. The extent to which he is willing to be directive is related, in most cases, to his approach to his specialty: the organic psychiatrist will be directive frequently, the dynamic psychiatrist rarely. Even though the patient may later feel animosity about the advice, as Virginia Woolf did,[1] no particular legal issues are involved. Legal issues are raised when the psychiatrist is asked either to determine a patient's mental state to justify a procedure to prevent progeny (sterilization procedures on male or female) or to certify that a patient's mental state is such that the continuation of an existing pregnancy is a hazard to the mother and that accordingly an abortion is indicated.

STERILIZATION

Sterilization procedures, male or female, are categorized as *1.* eugenic, *2.* therapeutic, and *3.* sterilization of convenience. Eugenic sterilizations are performed usually on unwilling subjects who the state believes would be unfit parents because of mental disability. Therapeutic sterilizations are performed on willing subjects—the patient must give consent to the procedure—because medical opinion indicates that further pregnancies may endanger the life of the mother. Sterilizations of convenience are performed on eager subjects who believe that this will be the most certain or the most satisfactory method of birth control.

EUGENIC STERILIZATION

Eugenic sterilization, usually against the will of the subject, is performed under authority of state law. The movement for enactment of enabling statutes had its greatest impetus during the early years of this century, when the concepts of human perfectibility and an ideal society seemed possible of attainment, partly under the influence of ideas then held concerning heredity and other causes of mental illness, which were oversimplified. Because compulsory surgery—like the lobotomy forced on a patient under authority of the state—smacks of authoritarianism, is difficult to reconcile with Anglo-Saxon ideas of the preservation of individual rights, and has connotations associated with Hitlerian ideas of preservation of racial purity and sacrifice for the state, such sterilization has been losing popularity, although the laws of 28 states provide for eugenic sterilization of the feeble-minded, insane, sexual deviates and habitual criminals.[2]

A bill introduced in Michigan in 1897 was defeated, and a Pennsylvania bill of 1905 vetoed; Indiana, in 1907, became the first state to enact a compulsory sterilization law, in response to recently devised methods.

Until the end of the nineteenth century sterilization was impractical because castration, the only method known at the time, caused undesirable changes in secondary sexual characteristics and was considered too radical an operation to use for eugenic reasons. In the last decade of the century, however, Dr. Harry C. Sharpe of the Indiana State Reformatory developed a method of sterilizing males (vasectomy), and at about the same time the now standard method of sterilizing females (salpingectomy) was developed in France.[3]

The vasectomy consists of making skin incisions in the scrotum and interrupting each *vas deferens*, the duct leading from the testicle to the ejaculatory duct. It is a simpler procedure than the salpingectomy, for the female, which requires an abdominal incision and the interruption of the fallopian tubes, down which the egg must travel to the uterus. "Neither interferes with the desire for sexual intercourse or with its gratification."[4]

Challener tells of the controversy about the sterilization bill, entitled a "bill for the prevention of idiocy," which the Pennsylvania legislature passed in 1905. It authorized a surgeon "to perform such operation for the prevention of procreation as shall be deemed safest and most effective." In vetoing the bill, the governor noted the attractive title of the bill but stated his belief that it empowered the surgeon to "cut the heads off the inmates" if it was his belief that this was the safest and most effective method of preventing procreation.[5] Indiana enacted the first compulsory sterilization act in 1907, but this and other acts prior to 1925 were eventually declared unconstitutional.

In 1925, statutes in Michigan and Virginia were upheld by the highest courts of those states, and the United States Supreme Court, in the famous case of *Buck* vs *Bell* in 1927, upheld the Virginia law.

Justice Oliver Wendell Holmes, the Yankee from Olympus who had never forgotten his days as a soldier in the Civil War, and who carried his patriotism to the point of making the United States the beneficiary of his will, believed that the sacrifice of an individual forced to give up his opportunity for procreation and to submit to a surgical invasion of his scrotum (or her abdomen) was no greater than the sacrifices that the government requires of its soldiers during war, also for the common good. He stated that the case law upholding the right of states to enforce compulsory vaccination law against smallpox by analogy could apply to those who would not be "vaccinated" against another communicable disease, pregnancy.

The Holmes decision was based on the assumption that the defects were hereditary in the absence of any scientific evidence challenging this theory, and on the precedent of the Massachusetts compulsory vaccination law (which, however, provided that those who "should deem it important that vaccination should not be performed" had merely to pay a fine of five dollars to escape the procedure).

It has been argued that the Massachusetts vaccination statute and the Virginia sterilization statute are not analogous because "so far as concerns liberty there would appear to be a real difference between assessing a fine and compelling submission. . . ." Moreover, the scientific findings relating the prevention of smallpox with vaccination are more conclusive than the highly controverted claim that mental disorders are largely hereditary.

Justice Holmes also made another analogy in *Buck v. Bell*. It was to the effect that if the nation can call upon its best citizens to sacrifice their lives in time of war, the nation should be able to ask a lesser sacrifice of those who are already a burden to it. This analogy has been criticized on the ground that there is "a necessity and an urgency that causes us to sacrifice men in self-defense which is wholly lacking in the case of eugenic sterilization."[6]

Twenty-eight states now have so-called involuntary sterilization laws, but in two of these (Minnesota and Vermont) the consent of the subject must be obtained. In all these states, the laws apply to patients in state institutions, and in six of them to persons outside institutions. The laws apply to the mentally deficient, the mentally ill, and—in 18 states—epileptics. Some of these laws also apply to "hereditary criminals" (twelve states), sex offenders, and even syphilitics.

The American Neurological Association Committee for the Investigation of Eugenic Sterilization concluded that compulsory sterilization could not be advocated on the basis of the present state of scientific knowledge of hereditary mental conditions. Certainly provisions for the compulsory sterilization of epileptics are outdated in the light of current medical opinion.

When considered in the light of recent scientific thinking the validity of sterilization for eugenic purposes is certainly open to serious questioning. In evaluating the advisability of compulsory sterilization it is important to keep in mind that mental illness and epilepsy have shown an increased response to medical treatment. It is also important to remember that though there is some relationship between heredity and mental deficiency, it has been estimated that about 89 per cent of inheritable mental deficiency is passed on by individuals not themselves deficient. At the present time there is no way of ascertaining who these normal carriers are. Thus, if it were possible to sterilize collectively all the feeble-minded, their number in the following generation would be cut down only about 11 per cent. It has been asserted that at present there is no scientific basis for any plan to eliminate completely the problem of mental deficiency.[7]

Figures compiled by the Human Betterment Association for Voluntary Sterilization show a steady decline in the number of institutionalized patients sterilized yearly since 1950, when the figure was over 1,500, to the early '60's, when the figure was less than 500 and falling yearly. They also show a change in the ratio of the categories sterilized: for the fifteen year period from 1946 to 1961, 52% of those sterilized were mentally deficient, 44% were mentally ill, and 4% were listed as "others," a category including epileptics, perverts, and degenerates. In 1961, the comparable figures were 71% mentally deficient, 21% mentally ill, and 7% "others," indicating perhaps the more favorable view of state institution superintendents on the prognosis of the mentally ill in their care.[8]

Morton Birnbaum, who has a degree both in law and medicine, has described another type of eugenic sterilization—the detention of a patient until she is too old to reproduce—as "institutional sterilization."[9]

Where eugenic surgical sterilization is not practiced because the medical staff believes that the law does not allow it, or because they do not approve of it because of medical, social, or religious beliefs, there may be a question of whether patients who are now involuntarily institutionalized for life would be discharged if surgical sterilization were performed; therefore, the issue then becomes the question of whether the eugenic sterilization is being accomplished by institutionalization, that is by segregation, rather than by surgery.

He describes the case of a mentally deficient girl who had been a patient in a New York state institution since early adolescence. At the age of 20, she was discharged on probation and a position was obtained for her at a nursing home; three months later, she became pregnant and was returned to the institution. The author saw her four days post-partum and comments that "the institution now has two patients where before it had one."

As the New York state mental institution will not perform eugenic surgical sterilization, she may be involuntarily eugenically institutionally sterilized by the state in spite of the fact that her own mental status does not require any further institutionalization. This may be done primarily because of a belief that discharge probably will result in sexual exploitation that in turn probably will result in future illegitimate pregnancies.

Birnbaum is not necessarily advocating wider use of surgical sterilization; he is advocating improvement of public mental institutions, adequate treatment, rehabilitation and follow-up to minimize the necessity of resorting to any type of sterilization, plus consideration of surgical sterilization as an alternative to "institutional sterilization," if this seems an advance. The Human Betterment Association for Voluntary Sterilization advocates wider use of sterilization for the mentally deficient as an alternative to custodial care during years when conception is possible. Bass has pointed out the difficulties in teaching consistent use of contraception to the mental defective. "Surgical birth control, which has been proven acceptable to many who are unwilling or unable to use temporary methods of contraception, would appear to be the most suitable method for mentally deficient persons." Laws that prohibit marriage for the retarded, aimed at preventing both the birth of children to those unable to care for them and the transmission of hereditary conditions, could be replaced by more liberal laws allowing marriage of sterilized persons.[10]

Surgical sterilization as an alternative to institutional sterilization is an elective procedure and not entirely comparable to the enforced sterilization of the insane, the criminal, and the sexually deviated, although in each the threat of continued incarceration may be the pressure that turns an apparently voluntary into an involuntary operation. The two can be distinguished on the bases of the potential ability to use contraception and that the intention in surgically sterilizing the defective is not punitive. Deserving consideration is the always troublesome legal question of the ability of the mental defective to give consent to a procedure that may be difficult for him to comprehend.

Intrauterine contraceptive devices have been suggested as alternative to "surgical birth control." The low cost and ease of insertion of these devices may make them preferable to the salpingectomy; but when used by the mentally defective as alternative to continued in-

stitutionalization, the questions of possible duress and the validity of
the consent of the defective need consideration once again.

THERAPEUTIC STERILIZATION

The indication for therapeutic sterilization is danger to the life
of the mother from an additional pregnancy. Since any therapeutic
sterilization would be performed only after the patient and spouse had
both signed a written consent to the procedure, there is no real distinction between therapeutic and voluntary sterilization, except in two
states—Connecticut and Utah—where voluntary sterilization is prohibited. In these two states, voluntary sterilization can be performed
only when there is a therapeutic basis.

STERILIZATION OF CONVENIENCE

Virginia in 1962 became the first state to pass a voluntary sterilization law, but this gives legal sanction only to the existing practice,
which is to perform sterilizing operations on consenting adults when
the physician agrees that the operation is desirable. The main effect
of the Virginia statute was to make it clear that such indications for
sterilization as poor economic condition, too many children, and other
socioeconomic factors are valid.[11] Before the passage of this law, there
was probably no legal problem concerning voluntary sterilization either
in Virginia or in all the other states (with the exception of the two cited
above). The AMA pointed this out in 1961: "Until declared illegal by
the legislature or the courts in the physician's state, nontherapeutic
sterilization is largely a matter of individual conscience."[12]

Therapeutic sterilization concerns forensic medicine more than
forensic psychiatry, except for the considerations that these procedures
—because they involve such highly charged emotional areas as body
image, ability to procreate, and relationship of husband to wife—may
have more psychiatric sequelae than other surgical procedures. Dr.
Merlin H. Johnson believes that vasectomy is often a factor leading
to hospitalization for mental illness and notes that reasons given for
the procedure are often invalid. He cites one operation performed on a
man whose wife was 52 years old and another on a man of 53 whose
wife had had a hysterectomy 25 years earlier.[13]

In a recent State of Washington case, the plaintiff claimed negligence on the part of the physician in testing for viable sperm after the
operation and claimed mental anguish caused by the birth of a baby
after the operation as a factor in damages. The court ruled that the
birth of a normal, healthy offspring could not be considered a damaging
event.[14]

Birnbaum has pointed out that this is an area of law where decisions—to or not to allow a sterilization procedure—are in reality made by formal or informal tribunals composed of medical men, rather than by judicial tribunals composed of law men. The decisions are theoretically primarily medical, based on necessarily vague legal guidelines.[15] If a woman who has had four children desires to have a salpingectomy or her husband wishes a vasectomy, the surgeon will be guided by the policy of his hospital. A Catholic hospital may oppose the procedure, a proprietary hospital may allow it freely, and most hospitals will be guided by rules concerning age of the woman, number of surviving children and other somewhat arbitrary criteria. The Committee of Human Reproduction of the American Medical Association in 1965 issued a statement on surgical sterilization.[16]

Medical opinions concerning proper indications for surgical sterilization of either sex range all the way from absolutely none at all to a list which includes the following: (1) afflictions of a hereditary nature involving previous offspring of the marriage or, in some instances, the hereditary involvement of one or both actual or potential parents; (2) conditions in the mother that may be aggravated by repeated pregnancies; (3) physical, mental, or emotional defects which may seriously impair the functioning of either husband or wife as an adequate parent or which cause the physician to conclude that parenthood at any future time would be hazardous or both; and (4) multiparity to a degree affecting adversely the woman's health or well-being.

That state laws regarding sterilization are not only different, but have been interpreted differently, has added to the confusion regarding the legal status of sterilization. Likewise concern has been expressed regarding the possibility of untoward after-effects of a psychological nature, particularly if remarriage or death of already-born children creates a desire for additional offspring. Hence, it would seem desirable for the medical profession to arrive at a consensus regarding sterilization that would provide solid ground for performing it where it appears indicated. At the same time, the development and improvement of present methods and the advent of new methods of contraception should, if properly understood and widely applied, serve to diminish the need for permanent contraception by means of surgical sterilizing procedures.

ABORTION

The problem of abortion comes into legal psychiatry more clearly. Because the death of the fetus *in utero* is considered a serious matter, abortions are allowed only when medical necessity is shown; and as progress has been made in medicine's ability to take care of the mother —making it more difficult for a doctor to certify that an abortion is required on the basis of heart, kidney or other organ function—the psychiatrist has been increasingly asked to certify the need for abortion on grounds of mental health.

There is a difference, on the legal responsibilities of doctors, between standard texts that take a strict view concerning abortion, and doctors who have expressed themselves in recent years to the effect that within the framework of existing laws the physician can widen the scope of the indications for abortion. Formerly, for instance, it was not considered an indication for abortion that there was a possibility (the figure is sometimes given roughly as a 30% possibility, although the estimates have ranged widely) of a malformed infant because the mother had contracted German measles during the first trimester. Now doctors who formerly refused to abort on this indication do so freely. The increasingly liberal view about indications for abortion is not the result of new statutes or case law or even new scientific information about the indications and validity of abortion; instead, it seems to represent the pressure of public opinion, the willingness of the medical profession to go along with that opinion, and the reluctance of public authorities to question the reasoning and judgment of reputable physicians practicing in recognized hospitals.

The texts and handbooks clearly state that abortions are justified only when the life of the mother is in danger. Says Long in *The Physician and the Law:*

In general, the right of a physician to perform an abortion is restricted to cases where continuance of pregnancy would constitute an imminent danger to the health or life of the mother. In some states abortion constitutes a felony and in others it is a misdemeanor. . . . The right to perform a therapeutic abortion is based on necessity in each case. Necessity is a complete defense both at common law and under the statute. . . . The defense of necessity applies only to cases where imminent danger to the mother is based on causes connected with delivery. . . . The defense of necessity is not available if the abortion was procured to prevent the mother from committing suicide. . . . Some statutes permit an abortion if a physician advised that it was necessary for the purpose of preserving life.[17]

Moritz and Stetler in their *Handbook of Legal Medicine* say:

All states have statutes which provide, in substance, that the performance of an abortion without therapeutic justification is unlawful. . . . State abortion statutes are variously worded, but most of them provide that the act is not criminal when the abortion is necessary to save or to preserve the life of the woman . . . or advised by physicians (usually two) as being necessary to preserve the life of the woman.[18]

Preserving the life of the woman implies either a medical condition, such as heart disease, kidney disease, hypertension, tuberculosis, where continuation of the pregnancy would probably lead to death, or a psychiatric condition, such as the probability of suicide, if the pregnancy is not terminated. As organic medical indications for abortion have been disappearing (in response to advanced methods of hospital care and anesthetic and surgical technics), the psychiatrist has been increasingly called on to certify that because the patient has had previous instability or psychotic illness, is depressed and is threatening suicide, continuation of the pregnancy constitutes a danger to the mother. The doctor advising an abortion may be an obstetrician who feels that because a mother is unmarried, or extremely young (increasingly, pregnancies are occurring in those under 15), or has been the victim of an alleged rape, this procedure should be carried out. But because he cannot certify that this would be a lifesaving procedure for the mother, and because he is unwilling to put his own head on the block and give his own opinion that the patient is so psychiatrically ill that her life is in danger, he seeks the certification of psychiatrists so that the hospital record on this matter will be in order. Many reputable psychiatrists—probably most reputable psychiatrists—do not believe that pregnancy will probably lead to suicide,[19] even when the threat is made; and psychiatrists are aware that one reason for the threat of suicide may be the knowledge that this is the password that opens the door to the psychiatric certification that is being sought. Most psychiatrists, therefore, certify abortions very rarely. Some, on the other hand—possessed of such nonlegal motives as the belief that the abortion laws should be modernized, or that an abortion is not a very serious procedure, or that unwanted babies should not be brought into the world, or that an adolescent girl should not be put through the rigors of childbirth, or, perhaps, merely of the desire to cooperate with the referring obstetrician, who may be on the staff of his hospital and a productive source of referrals—these may allow their consciences flexibility enough to permit them to certify that a suicide is "certainly" in the offing.

At the same time, more and more nonpsychiatrist physicians are stretching the criteria for abortions, knowing that no real medical or psychiatric indications exist, but acting in the belief that the abortion laws are too restrictive and that enforcement officials do not inspect the internal affairs of reputable hospitals to question the basis for abortions by reputable medical personnel. If a mother has had German measles in the first trimester of her pregnancy and has a 30% chance of having a baby with a congenital deformity, the life of the mother is not threatened. Yet abortions for rubella are increasing.[20]

Niswander and Klein analyzed the reasons for the certification of 500 abortions performed at two teaching hospitals between 1943 and 1964. They concluded that the results showed a more liberal physician attitude in recent years towards therapeutic abortion. The incidence per 1,000 deliveries was 8.4 in the 1960–64 period, double that of earlier periods.

Over the years, changes in medical indications included decreases in the percentage of therapeutic abortions done for tuberculosis and cardiovascular disease; an increase in the proportion done for rubella, particularly in epidemic years; and an almost linear increase in those done for psychogenic reasons. A marked rise was evident in the percentage of girls under 20 receiving therapeutic abortions, and the percentage of married patients decreased from 93.3% during 1943–49 to 58.9% during 1960–64.

Other findings included the following: (1) psychogenic reasons were greatest among girls under 20 and women over 39 and among Jewish women compared with Protestants and Catholics; (2) among the unmarried patients, 93.7% of abortions were for psychic indications; and (3) the affluent woman was much more likely to be aborted than the indigent woman.

The analysis indicates, said the authors, that "a significant proportion of our abortions would not fit comfortably into most statutes on legal abortion." They pointed out, for instance, that psychogenic abnormality would rarely seem to increase the risk of death in a gravid patient. They believe that "changes are occurring in the attitudes of doctors, and, by implication, in the attitudes of society at large toward therapeutic abortion. . . . If good law represents the opinion of the majority, the time for reconsideration of the laws governing therapeutic abortion has arrived."[21]

A New York City study showed a 65% decrease in therapeutic abortions over the 20 years from 1943 to 1962. It also showed that therapeutic abortions among the white population were more than five times those among the nonwhites and 26 times those among the Puerto Rican population. Variations in the frequency of therapeutic abortions among hospital categories has persisted. The frequency was five times as high in the proprietary hospital (6.3:1,000 live births) as in the municipal hospitals (1.2:1,000), while the figure in voluntary nonproprietary hospitals was between these two extremes (3.2:1,000). Within the voluntary nonproprietary hospitals, the incidence differed between the private services (3.6:1,000) and the central services (1.9:1,000). Dr. Edwin M. Gold, reporting on the survey, said that the differences between hospital categories, as well as among ethnic groups, are determined, apparently, partly by general community attitudes, the relative economic status of the patients, and their cultural and social mores. "The most influential factors are probably the attitude of individual physicians and hospitals toward therapeutic abortions in connection with the greater sophistication, in general, of the white population and its opinion regarding appropriate family size."

In contrast to the sharp drop in therapeutic abortions over the 20-year period, there was only a 19% drop in such abortions based on mental disorders, and the psychiatric indication for abortion remained the major ground for certification throughout the period.[22]

Dr. Robert G. Hall, of Obstetrics and Gynecology at the Columbia University College of Physicians and Surgeons, has reported a strikingly higher incidence of therapeutic abortions on private services compared to ward services, and reported figures for Sloane Hospital for Women for the period 1951 to 1960 as one abortion per 55 deliveries for private patients and 1:224 for ward patients. Dr. Hall has called for the liberalization of state laws "to permit the indications for abortion which accepted medical practice has already legitimized," and has said that since it is the obstetricians who violate existing abortion laws, it is they "who should seek their renovation."[23]

The Association for Human Abortion calls for the right to certify therapeutic abortions in these situations not covered by present laws: when the health of the mother, but not necessarily her life, is threatened; where the continuation of the pregnancy constitutes a severe handicap to a chronic mentally or physically ill woman; where physical or mental abnormality in the newborn is likely; where there has been rape or incest; or when pregnancy occurs in a child under 16 years.[24]

Those who call for a more liberal attitude on abortion point to the estimated million or 1,500,000 criminal abortions performed in the United States each year, in comparison with a mere 18,000 legal therapeutic abortions. (Estimates run from 8,000 to 18,000.)

A recent magazine article provides an "abortion fact sheet":

A million illegal abortions are performed annually, mostly on women who are married and have several children. Experts say thousands of women die, but the cause is concealed.

Legal abortions are permitted in hospitals for 8,000 to 12,000 women a year whose lives are "endangered" by pregnancy. Many doctors say that under existing state laws most of these abortions are illegal. They want to have the laws liberalized.

Poorer women are the main victims in this tragic situation. They find it much harder to get legal abortions and fall prey to butchery. A great many try to abort themselves.

Competent illegal abortions are performed in almost every US city; prices are often high. Many women journey to Mexico and Puerto Rico, where abortions are illegal but cheaper. In Japan, cheap abortions are obtained legally.

The Catholic Church opposes liberalizing present abortion laws. This has strained its relations with other religions in such places as California, where the debate is bitter.[25]

The American Law Institute in 1959 proposed liberalized state laws on abortion, although one authority has estimated that the changes it recommends would not even double the present small number of therapeutic abortions: "it would merely legitimize them." Therapeutic abortions would be allowed if doctors thought there was great risk that continuance of a pregnancy would gravely impair the mental or physical health of a mother—thus putting increased demands on the psychiatrist to make this determination—and also if the pregnancy resulted from rape or incest, or if there was significant risk that the child might have a grave physical or mental defect.[26]

This definition lowers the standard from that now in use, danger to the life of the mother, to impairment of the health of the mother. Even this liberalized standard would not help the million women in the United States who each year obtain illegal abortions for entirely nonmedical reasons. These are the women whose health and welfare are threatened because they have abortions in places other than hospitals. To serve the demands of this group of women, it has been suggested that the decision to abort should be based entirely on personal reasons without any consideration of medical factors. Says the organizer of the Society for Humane Abortion: "Who wants to go before a board for an abortion? It should be a private matter between a doctor and a woman, just like any other surgery."[27]

In other parts of the world—such as Japan and Eastern Europe—abortions can be secured simply, inexpensively, and legally. Hungary in 1964 had 218,700 registered abortions for 132,100 births, a ratio of 166 abortions to 100 births. It was estimated that the average Hungarian woman has had more than three abortions by the end of her fertile span. In Rumania, women may obtain abortions simply on request at hospitals and factory clinics, giving no reason and not being required to give their names. The patient is allowed to go home after two hours; the physician is not allowed to perform more than ten abortions a day.[28]

The United States, with an estimated three of every ten pregnancies terminating in abortion, is faced with the decision whether to yield to pressure from mothers and doctors to bring this group of cases into the area of reputable hospital service.[29] On one side is the desire for good medical care for women who will seek bad medical care if they have no alternative. In the enlightened society of the future, says the president of the New York County Medical Society, "a mother's right to determine how many children she desires will be guaranteed by the Bill of Rights, and no unwanted children will be brought into the world."[30] On the other side is the view embodied in the statutes of all United States jurisdictions that a life *in utero* is protected by the law, and that the termination of the life *in utero* is the crime of feticide, except when the life of the mother is in danger. Pflum has stated that an answer to the argument that illegal abortions are so often fatal to the mother is the reminder that "abortions, legal and illegal, are one hundred percent fatal to the lives in utero."[31] Sonne suggests that even when a mentally deranged woman asks her therapist to help her obtain an abortion, the feticidal wish should not be seen as coherent or valid but rather as "not only irrational, but irretrievably destructive of life as well. . . . Feticide is a renunciation of the roots of reason," and leads to a "permanent denial of the possibilities of psychotherapy if it is sanctioned by the therapist."[32]

When the AMA's House of Delegates met in Philadelphia in November, 1965, it received a report from its Board of Trustees transmitting the recommendation of the Committee on Human Reproduction to liberalize abortion laws by permitting therapeutic abortion if pregnancy constitutes a threat to the mother's health (rather than a threat to her life).[33] The Committee on Human Reproduction recommended that abortion be permitted when there is a substantial risk that the physical or mental health of the mother would be gravely impaired if she continued to carry the child, as well as when there is a substantial risk of the child's having grave physical or mental defects or when the pregnancy resulted from rape or incest. However, a legislation committee considering this recommendation reported that it had received conflicting testimony on the justification and necessity of abortion under these circumstances. "The problem is essentially one for resolution by each state through action of its own legislature. . . . It is not appropriate at this time for the AMA to recommend enactment of legislation in this matter for all states." The vote of the House of Delegates finally was to defer action on a new stand concerning abortion and in the meantime merely to confer with lawyers, clergymen, sociologists, legislators, and government administrators on the subject.[34]

The problem of abortion is not too different from that of euthanasia. In each case, a life is at stake that may have less value than an ordinary life. Should the traditional medical—and moral—value of preserving life be abandoned? Should the determination of life or death—which has always been considered a legal determination—be placed in the hands of a doctor or a board of doctors? If the criteria for securing an abortion are broadened to encompass any substantial risk to the physical or mental health of a mother, would there be any limit to the number of abortions that could be secured under this formula?

If the criteria for securing an abortion are considerably liberalized, or if, as it has been proposed, the crime of feticide is wiped from the books, the result will be changes in basic attitudes towards life and sexual behavior. As the AMA House of Delegates has recognized, any decision to alter established law on this subject is obviously the responsibility of the legislatures that placed on the books the present restrictions on abortion. The present tendency of the obstetrician to anticipate changes in legislation by taking it on himself to liberalize the indications for therapeutic abortion in advance of legislative action seems neither wise nor helpful. The long-term effects on American life of a changed approach to the problem of abortion seem to be matters for debate in state legislatures rather than for extralegal determination by obstetricians and other physicians.

CHAPTER 12

Mental Suffering and Traumatic Neurosis

WHEN a broken leg is the subject of a legal action for damages, the plaintiff has the task of proving in court that his injury resulted from the negligence or intentional injury of the defendant. If the case goes his way, he will have the opportunity to present evidence to show the extent of his disability and the duration of his incapacity, so that the court can determine the amount of damages he should be awarded, and for this purpose the testimony of witnesses and records, including doctors' reports, hospital charts and such tangible evidence as roentgenograms, will be admitted. The plaintiff will then itemize his expenses and his loss of income; the guilty defendant will be assessed for these, and, in addition, sometimes for that nebulous effect of trauma, the mental or emotional suffering that the plaintiff experienced. The principle that the mental suffering that accompanies physical injury is compensable is firmly established and time-honored.

In another group of cases, the plaintiff has experienced mental or emotional suffering—fright, humiliation, or anxiety—without any physical injury and without any accompanying physical signs or symptoms. Nineteenth-century courts, in both England and America, would not allow damages in these. In a famous often-cited case of a century ago, Lord Wensleydale stated: "mental pain or anxiety, the law cannot value and does not pretend to redress when the unlawful act causes that alone."[1] One eminent authority, Prosser, says that in such a case no damages lie, because "physical injury" or "physical consequences" must be shown to support recovery.

Where the defendant's negligence causes only mental disturbance without accompanying physical injury or physical consequences, there has been general agreement that there can be no recovery. The temporary emotion of fright, with no physical harm, is so evanescent a thing, so easily counterfeited, and usually so trivial, that the courts have been unwilling to protect the plaintiff against mere negligence. . . .[2]

93

FOUR BASES FOR LIABILITY

But when a case comes to court involving the effects of fright or humiliation without physical impact on the person—perhaps the emotion he experienced was the result of an explosion in which he sustained no injuries, of a false death notice sent as a "practical" joke, of witnessing an assault on another person, or even of physical contact so slight as a kiss or an undesired hug—the courts, as the law evolved, have found four bases for granting damages for mental pain and suffering.

The first is the oldest—so old that the line of cases has been traced back to 1348. *Evil intent and malice* make for liability in cases where mere negligence would not be enough to support damages. Particularly in cases of unprovoked assault, courts will grant damages for mental pain or suffering although the assault missed its mark or even —during this century—although the assault was successful but the plaintiff, who was frightened and brings suit, was not the victim but only an observing bystander. The 1348 case involved an innkeeper's wife at whom a guest at the inn threw a hatchet.[3] Although she dodged it successfully, she brought suit—or rather, this being the reign of Edward III, her husband brought suit on account of her cause of action—and won. The names have not survived and we know the parties only by initial; the case is *I de S et ux.* vs *W de S.*

The second basis is also time-honored. Just as courts have held that certain categories of helpless individuals get special consideration from the law, other groups have the obligation to conform to stricter-than-average standards. The two groups that have been singled out to abide by particularly high standards are providers of *public transportation* and *public lodging*—common carriers and innkeepers. In exchange for the privilege of dealing with the entire public, they owe special duties to the entire public. Railroads have been held liable when their employee called a passenger a "deadbeat and swindler"[4] or when a lady passenger was the subject of an "indecent proposal."[5] The same principle has gradually been enlarged to include owners of other premises which cater to the public—theaters, amusement parks, circuses, office buildings. Says Prosser: "There is no very visible reason why the same result might not be reached, in a proper case, as to any storekeeper; but in the instances which have arisen thus far recovery has been denied, possibly because the defendant's conduct was not sufficiently extreme."[6]

The third basis for recovery for mental suffering without physical trauma goes back to only the 1890's, when courts for the first time acknowledged that *miscarriages*—and in the intervening years that *other physical conditions*, such as heart attacks, strokes, and even ulcers

—might result from emotional causes. *Dulieu vs White and Sons,*[7] an English case, is one of the historic precedents on the subject of legal liability for psychic stimuli. The plaintiff alleged that on July 20, 1900, she was pregnant and working behind the bar of her husband's public house, when the defendant negligently drove a pair of horse vans into the tavern and frightened her so badly that she suffered a nervous shock and, as a consequence, a miscarriage.

Said Justice Kennedy, in answer to the argument that the driver could not anticipate that his precipitate action would lead to all the trouble that followed:

It may be admitted that the plaintiff, as regards the personal injuries, would not have suffered exactly as she did, if she had not been pregnant at the time; and no doubt the driver of the defendant's horses could not anticipate that she was in this condition. But what does that fact matter? If a man is negligently run over or otherwise negligently injured, it is no answer to the sufferer's claim for damages that he would have suffered less injury, or no injury at all, if he had not had an unusually thin skull or an unusually weak heart.

The test is risk of injury to the average person, and even though the traumatic stimulus is only psychic and the defendant is unaware of the plaintiff's vulnerability, if the average such plaintiff would run a risk of a similar unfortunate result under similar circumstances, then the injury is compensable. In the American case that sets forth the doctrine of psychic stimulus ten years before Judge Kennedy's decision, the defendant knew that the plaintiff was pregnant; his assault was not on the plaintiff but on her family servants in her presence. Her fright and emotional state led to a miscarriage, and the court found the defendant liable for this consequence of his actions.[8]

The fourth basis for recovery on the ground of psychic stimulus is grounded on concepts of modern psychiatry and psychosomatic medicine, although Goodrich, writing in 1922,[9] cited Charles Darwin's observations of the physiologic effect of fright in animals rather than relying on Freudian theory. According to this basis, transient or evanescent emotional states still cannot be alleged as compensable, but many of the *emotional effects of psychic stimuli* might be more disabling and more permanent than courts had previously considered, and the *physiologic response of the individual* might be more subject to description in court—in terms of such phenomena as blood pressure, hormonal response to fear, effect of emotions on processes such as digestion—than had been thought previously. Courts now, at least in some jurisdictions could see that besides the gross manifestations of psychic trauma —miscarriages, heart attacks, strokes—there could be more subtle manifestations, such as ulcers or even anxieties and other neurotic symptoms, which were nonetheless capable of legal proof.

MOOD OF THE COURT

But in spite of four bases for recovery for mental suffering unaccompanied by such physical symptoms as fractures and concussions, the general mood of the court has been reluctance to award damages, although a few cases in recent years indicate that the reluctance may be abating. What is behind the court's resistance to dealing with mental suffering on the same basis as it does with physical suffering, particularly since some jurists have pointed out that it is the same brain that experiences the suffering in each case?

Prosser has stated how reluctant courts were to inquire into any mental phenomenon, whether in negligent or intentional damage or in contracts, wills, marriage and even criminal responsibility. In 1467, Chief Justice Brian had opined, "The thought of man should not be tried, for the devil himself knoweth not the thought of man."[10] Two centuries later, courts still felt that the tangible evidence of documents and actions could be the basis of a rational system of justice, but that the vague evidence of intentions, thoughts, concepts and conclusions could not. Courts then would not permit evidence of a man's knowledge, belief or intentions, on the ground that these are entirely subjective and "cannot be known." In 1681, an English court ruled that the defendant in a contract case could not present evidence of his intention. "Upon this the plaintiff demurred and had judgment, for it appears that the fact was voluntary, and his intention and knowledge are not traversable; they cannot be known."[11] As time went on, however, courts began to delve into beliefs, knowledge, understanding and intent; the idea that mutual consent based on mutual understanding must be present before contracts and quasicontractual agreements (such as marriage) came into effect became one of the themes interwoven into all the aspects of jurisprudence.

Even after courts were united in their willingness to delve into thought, as in determining the intention of a party to a contract, they were still unwilling to delve into feeling. These questions were considered too nebulous to deal with in the practical-minded courtroom, and courts stated repeatedly that if they granted recovery for "mental suffering" in cases involving shock or fright without physical impact, then they would be flooded by litigation involving issues with which the courts were not prepared to deal. "If the right of recovery in this class of cases should be once established," a New York court stated in 1896, "it would naturally result in a flood of litigation in cases where the injury complained of may be easily feigned without detection,"[12] and the following year a Massachusetts court similarly held that recovery should be denied in a mental suffering case for fear that it "would open a wide door for unjust claims, which could not successfully be met."[13] Says Morris, "The courts feared that by faking physical injury, or falsely attributing it to emotional upset, plaintiffs might impose on courts and defendants."[14]

Even at this stage of the development of law, if physical contact or physical damage could be the peg on which an action for damages could hang, a court would sometimes be willing to compensate for injured feelings. To his famed dictum that "mental pain or anxiety, the law cannot value, and does not pretend to redress, when the unlawful act causes that alone," Lord Wensleydale immediately added: "Though, where a material damage occurs, and is connected with it, it is impossible a jury, in estimating it, should altogether overlook the feelings of the party interested." That courts are becoming more liberal than they were in Lord Wensleydale's day, a century ago, is indicated by some recent cases. In *Falzone* vs *Busch*, the New Jersey Supreme Court ruled that the plaintiffs could maintain a suit for damages from an automobile accident in which Mrs. Falzone was not struck but from which, she claimed, she suffered a disabling ailment by reason of her fright. The defendant's car struck Mr. Falzone, then veered across the road narrowly missing the parked car in which Mrs. Falzone was sitting. The Superior Court ruled that a decision of 1900 barring recovery for damages when there was no impact was controlling, but on appeal the higher court stated that the reasons for the 1900 ruling were no longer tenable and it was questionable if they ever were. And a New York Court has awarded $740,000 in damages for a death from a heart attack when a car cut across the decedent's lawn.[15]*

Three reasons have usually been given for the reluctance of courts to award damages for mental suffering. One is the difficulty of proving the injury or measuring the damages; mental suffering has sometimes been considered "too subtle and speculative to be capable of admeasurement by any standard known to the law."[16] A second is that the mental consequences of an act so vary with the individual concerned that they cannot be anticipated and lie outside the boundaries of any reasonable "proximate connection" with the act of the defendant. The third is the flood of litigation that might develop and the proba-

---

* The $740,000 award in *Caposella* vs *Kelley* was made under unusual circumstances. The defendant's lawyer had died four years before the trial; the award was made in default, and the defendant then alleged that she had not known of the hearing and consequently had not been represented in court. The award was later vacated. *Newsweek*, December 27, 1965, reported that the plaintiff's lawyer was preparing to go to trial again and that this case had again raised the question of whether fright or a similar shock can trigger a fatal attack in a person afflicted with heart disease.

bility that law would now be forced to look into questions that formerly had been considered matters of manners and social relationships.

Prosser answers all these arguments.[17] Concerning the difficulty in measuring mental suffering, he points out that although the physical pain of a broken leg is not easily assessed, courts are willing to assess it. In either case, as we have said, the pain is a mental phenomenon: "All pain is mental and centers in the brain. . . ." Concerning the alleged lack of "proximate connection" or causation between act and the mental or emotional disturbance, which would make the results of the act foreseeable to the defendant, Prosser says:

It is not difficult to discover in the earlier opinions a distinctly masculine astonishment that any woman should ever be so silly as to allow herself to be frightened or shocked into a miscarriage. But medical science has recognized long since that not only fright and shock, but also grief, anxiety, rage and shame, are in themselves 'physical' injuries, in the sense that they produce well marked changes in the body, and symptoms that are readily visible to the professional eye. Such consequences are the normal, rather than the unusual, result of a threat of physical harm, and of many other types of conduct; and in any case, nearly all courts have discarded foreseeability as the sole criterion of legal cause.

Concerning the argument that extending reasons for recovery will loose a flood of litigation and make trivialities the bases for suits, he says (quoting the 1703 opinion of Chief Justice Holt): "It is the business of the law to remedy wrongs that deserve it, even at the expense of a 'flood of litigation,' and it is a pitiful confession of incompetence on the part of any court of justice to deny relief on such grounds. . . . 'If men will multiply injuries, actions must be multiplied; for every man that is injured ought to have his recompense.' "[18]

Although the psychiatrist concerns himself particularly with emotions and prides himself on his understanding of them, courts have never called in psychiatrists to evaluate mental suffering, whether it accompanied or did not accompany physical trauma, nor has the psychiatrist been called to testify how great a plaintiff's humiliation may be because of a slander or how great his anxiety because of danger. The courts perhaps feel that they are as competent to judge the reasonableness and the extent of such feelings without medical help. Magruder has cited some of the situations where courts feel competent to assess money damages for mental effects, and without the help of the psychiatrist.

The amorous railroad conductor who rained kisses upon the proper young school teacher cost his company $1,000 'compensatory' damages for her 'terror and anguish, her outraged feeling and insulted virtue, her mental humiliation and suffering.' It does not do to spit in another's face; this indignity, suffered by the plaintiff in the presence of a numerous company, was the basis of a judgment for $1,200. Two thousand dollars 'actual' damages for 'mental anguish and humiliation' was thought not excessive, where the hotel manager came to the plaintiff's room at night, and in vulgar and insulting terms accused her of being a common prostitute though in fact the gentleman who had come to visit her was none other than her lawfully wedded husband. Substantial sums have been recovered for false imprisonments, though the detention was of short duration and involved no damage other than annoyance and indignity. In many defamation cases where no special damages is alleged, the plaintiff recovers damages for mortification and outraged feelings. . . .[19]

However, in the past decades the plaintiff has increasingly claimed that the psychological effects of the trauma he received—and this trauma may have been directly physical or remotely psychological— have been more than evanescent feelings of fright and anguish and that they in fact constitute full-fledged psychiatric entities. Gradually, *traumatic neurosis*, *compensation neurosis*, and *malingering* began to appear in tort cases, and the psychiatrist to be called to testify about his knowledge of these conditions.

NEUROSES AND TORTS

The term *traumatic neurosis* or *traumatic psychoneurosis* has been surrounded by confusion. Psychiatrists have made the point that "traumatic neurosis" is not necessarily the same as "neurosis following trauma." Some have said that traumatic neurosis is a special entity with very specific diagnostic criteria; others have grouped a number of psychiatric conditions under the one heading. To add to the confusion, if there is a head trauma and a disturbed psychiatric condition results, this may be a traumatic neurosis but more probably represents an organic rather than a functional condition, and is therefore classified as an acute or a chronic brain syndrome.

Usdin has listed some terms that have been used as synonyms, although often incorrectly, for traumatic or posttraumatic neurosis or psychoneurosis[20]: *neurotic neurosis*, *neurosis following trauma*, *triggered neurosis*, *personal injury neurosis*, *occupational neurosis*, *stress reaction*, *combat fatigue*, *shell shock*, *compensation neurosis* and *secondary gain neurosis*. Considerable psychiatric attention first began to focus on the problem of the sudden development of neurosis after either stress or trauma during World War I, when symptoms of anxiety, fatigue, apathy, excitability, sleep disturbance, the development of phobias and other symptoms appeared in front line soldiers.

The name given to this condition, *shell shock*, indicates the nature of the trauma first implicated, the sudden onset of the condition, and the fact that the examining doctors felt that there was an organic etiology—the damage to the central nervous system from shell-blast concussions too close to the sufferer—that led to the symptoms. Later, it was observed that this phenomenon was not confined to front-line troops but was seen in soldiers never exposed to trauma or shell explosions, that often the onset was not sudden but insidious, that the victim sometimes had a previous history of neurotic problems, and that removal from the undesired situation (from the front lines in the case of a combat soldier, or from the Army itself in other cases) was sometimes the prerequisite to a cure. Says Kardiner in his chapter "Traumatic Neuroses of War,"[21] in the *American Handbook of Psychiatry*:

The "trauma" was thought to have given rise to some specific damage to the central nervous system. This notion was held, especially by neurologists, for a long time. There was much difficulty in establishing the actual damage, and even when demonstrated, the relation between the damage and the symptoms was never established. During World War I the issue was decided in favor of the so-called "functional" point of view.

Instead of the noncondemnatory or even approbatory titles that had been given to this condition—such as *combat neurosis, combat fatigue, shell shock, battle stress* or *stress reaction*—other less flattering terms came to be used. They cover both the battle situation and the homefront world of factory or office, where neurotic reactions may make dramatic appearances. The term *secondary gain neurosis* implies that the soldier or other victim has a purpose in being ill, the securing of some benefit, and that the illness may disappear either when the benefit is received or when the chance of gain—relief from a stressful situation or money damages—is eliminated from the situation. In purely peacetime situations, *personal injury neurosis, occupational neurosis,* and—the most commonly used of these terms—*compensation neurosis* carry the same kind of opprobrium, the implication that the patient is influenced by the desire for money damages or respite from a stressful situation. Many nonpsychiatrists, perhaps neurologists in particular, and a number of psychiatrists began to call many of these cases *malingering*, which implies conscious deception to avoid undesired situations or undesired work.

The confusion about nomenclature was only part of the problem. There was also confusion about etiology, as we have noted, and in addition there still is a gamut of medical views on diagnostic criteria, prognosis and recommended therapy for the condition. It is not surprising that the literature on the subject is complex and that courts as well as doctors are confused. But when all the categories of incapacity are boiled down to three main types—traumatic neurosis, compensation or triggered neurosis, and malingering—some of the difficulties disappear and, although complications still remain, at least the area becomes apparent where fruitful questions can be asked.

The first question is the relationship between mental pain and suffering (where psychiatric opinion is not sought by the courts) and mental pain and neurotic conditions (where the psychiatrist is acknowledged expert). Mental suffering and neurosis are not synonymous or even closely related. Mental suffering is any emotional distress; it is not in itself a physical condition, and it must usually be accompanied by some physical injury or contact, sometimes as slight as the conductor's kiss, before the courts will give damages. A neurosis is emotional, like mental suffering, but it has so developed that it fits some definite pattern described in the psychiatric nomenclature, whether the pattern is of depression and anxiety, or obsessive behavior, or hysterical symptoms. In its development to this point, the emotional turmoil has achieved the dignity of a medical diagnostic category.

As a starting point, there is the dictionary[22] definition of neurosis: "a functional disorder of the central nervous system usually manifested by anxiety, phobias, obsessions, or compulsions but frequently displaying signs of somatic disorder involving any of the bodily systems with or without other subjective or behavioral manifestations and having its most probable etiology in intrapsychic or interpersonal conflict. . . ." Psychiatrists are used to dealing with neurosis—it is their bread and butter, the backbone of their office practice—but the average neurosis does not give rise to a cause of legal action. When a patient shows symptoms of emotional distress, we usually ascribe them to the vicissitudes of his development, and although the patient may blame, and usually does, his mother, his father, and society in general, no one has made the legal claim that damages can be recovered from any one of this triumvirate. Even when the neurosis develops precipitately, rather than gradually, and an obvious external factor is involved— threat of loss of a job, a fall in the stock market, the birth of a baby, the death of a parent—unless the legal criterion is met of injury to the patient by someone who has the legal duty to deal with him less injuriously, there is no basis for recovery of damages. (One possible exception to this statement is in workmen's compensation law, but since different rules of liability apply, and since the award is an insurance payment rather than compensation for damages, tort cases and workmen's compensation cases can be differentiated.)

When a neurosis develops precipitately and there is such an obvious external factor as a hurricane, an automobile accident, a battle experience, a blow from a falling object or some other source of trauma, the condition graduates from the class of mere psychoneurosis and becomes a traumatic neurosis or a compensation neurosis. And in these cases there is a basis for recovery against a tortfeasor, or a claim against an insurer, or, as with a disabled soldier, the government.

Some authors use *traumatic neurosis* to describe any suddenly developing neurosis after trauma, even though the patient had shown symptoms of an unstable personality and even though the resulting neurosis is not clearly distinguishable from ordinary neuroses, such as anxiety state, hysteria, or obsessive-compulsive neurosis.

The first and most comprehensive approach to this subject, an article by Hubert Winston Smith, who is a graduate of both Harvard Medical School and Harvard Law School and represents the disciplines of law and forensic medicine, and Harry C. Solomon, a psychiatrist and neurologist, appeared in the *Virginia Law Review* in 1943 under the title "Traumatic Neuroses in Court."[23] It deals extensively with the topics of preexisting neurotic tendencies, but it does not limit the classification of traumatic neurosis to the development of a new neurosis in a hitherto mentally healthy person who has been subject to trauma. Instead, it deals with *traumatic* neurosis as if it were any neurosis—in most cases, according to these authors, an anxiety state, hysteria, obsessive compulsive neurosis, or (to use their "old-fashioned" phrase) a *neurasthenia*.

More recently, Thompson, in a study of 500 litigated cases,[24] uses *posttraumatic neurosis*, but, like Smith and Solomon, he does not deal with it as a distinct psychiatric entity. Instead, he lists seven run-of-the-mine neurotic conditions that happen to make their appearances after trauma: anxiety states in 81% of patients, hysteria in 15%, phobic neurosis in 5%, mixed (anxiety state and hysteria) in 4%, obsessive-compulsive neurosis in less than 1%, hypochondriasis in less than 1%, and a superimposed depression in 31%. (The figures total more than 100% because of multiple diagnoses.) The diagnosis of neurasthenia had been discarded in the 20 years since Smith and Solomon's study. Thompson concludes that "posttraumatic psychoneurosis is probably the most misunderstood condition that occurs in medicolegal cases," but his own use of the term *posttraumatic* rather than *traumatic*, and his failure to differentiate these conditions from *compensation neurosis*, only add to the misunderstanding.

In contrast to Smith and Solomon and to Thompson, what is the prevailing view of modern psychiatry on the reality of a separate entity, called *traumatic neurosis*, which is different from other neuroses found in the absence of trauma as well as a sequel to trauma?

The concept of *traumatic neurosis* is based on the psychiatric belief that just as a physical cause can produce physical disease, as an automobile accident may produce a fractured leg or a ruptured spleen, so can it produce a well-defined psychiatric disease—in a patient hitherto psychiatrically well and with no predisposition to psychiatric illness—

and that fright or stress alone, without physical trauma, can produce a similar result. The *American Handbook of Psychiatry* gives the original term as *Schreckneurose* ("terror neurosis").[25]

It is frequently found in such events as earthquakes, sea or military disasters, and mining catastrophes, but rarely in ordinary industrial or automobile accidents. It seems to be similar to the severe panic reactions described by Civil Defense authorities. Apparently, physical injury may be very slight or absent. Recurrent dreams, in which the patient relives the precipitating event in order to master the basic threat to life, are said to be common. Although the clinical picture may resemble an anxiety state, it is to be distinguished from a true hysteria. The patient may have no history of overt neurosis, and then the condition improves spontaneously. It is noteworthy that these panic states usually do not follow severe head injury in which there are unconsciousness and retrograde amnesia which may partially protect the patient; this fact reminds us that wounded soldiers seldom had severe anxiety states when brought into the hospital, as compared with their wound-free comrades.

The same source gives another definition of traumatic neurosis:

A specific and relatively infrequent panic state with predominant anxiety and hysteria. These characteristics are seen only in circumstances where there is extreme threat to life, as in holocausts, earthquakes, and major naval disasters, and not in industrial or automobile accidents. Here the word 'trauma' is used in the wider sense of physical and psychological factors causing harmful sequelae. The dynamics differ from those in ordinary hysteria, because the premorbid personality may be free from neurosis, and this may happen to anyone.

(The author, Brosin, does not explain why earthquakes can cause a traumatic neurosis while automobile and industrial accidents cannot.)

Harper characterizes traumatic neurosis by the symptoms of tremulousness, sweating, palpitations, crying, "and above all," very disturbing dreams.[26] He then adds: ". . . many symptoms . . . are part and parcel of this particular type of illness and no two of them are the same. It can extend into almost every facet of an individual's life: appetite, personal relationships, the ability to concentrate are all vulnerable." He finds a "very important" secondary reaction, the reversion to an almost child-like attitude with more and more reliance on others. He gives two contrasting cases as examples. In *Astle et al.* vs *Olmstead*,[27] plaintiff had been discharged from the army for a psychoneurosis induced by battle fatigue. His condition was said to have greatly improved, but after an automobile accident the nervousness returned. Expert testimony offered by the plaintiff asserted that the accident was the cause of the renewal of the nervous condition, and recovery was awarded. However, in *Davis* vs *Cleveland R. Co.*,[28] the plaintiff was caught in the folding doors of a bus; she offered evidence to show that although there were no bruises or wounds, the shock of this experience had caused a nervous disorder characterized by paralysis. Damages were not awarded.

No real basis for distinguishing between these two cases can be shown. The argument can be made that nervousness is a symptom of a traumatic neurosis and paralysis is not, and that recovery is allowed only for a traumatic neurosis and not for other sequelae of injuries. But the rationale behind this would still need to be clarified. If anything, the fact that in one case there was a preexisting psychiatric condition, the psychoneurosis induced by battle fatigue, would make it seem more fitting for the automobile victim to be denied damages and the bus passenger to be awarded them.

The questions surrounding traumatic neurosis can perhaps be boiled down to three—one medical, one legal, and one both. *First,* is there a clearly defined psychiatric entity, traumatic neurosis, which is distinguishable from other medical and psychiatric conditions—i.e., is it a clearly defined medical entity? *Second,* assuming that traumatic neurosis can be differentiated from all other psychiatric and medical consequences of trauma, should the patient who acquires this entity be compensated in the same way that he would be if he acquired a broken leg or a broken arm? *Third,* is there a factual basis for the legal concept that traumatic neuroses arise in mentally stable people—who, except for the traumatic incident, would have continued free of symptoms—while other psychiatric sequelae of tortious happenings that do not inflict physical injury occur to unstable individuals only?

At an American Psychiatric Association Round Table Meeting in 1960,[29] the five participants agreed that there *is* such an entity as traumatic neurosis. Much of the discussion of the evening concerned how this compensable condition can be differentiated from compensation neurosis and malingering. The term *compensation neurosis,* or Usdin's better *triggered neurosis,* is used to cover all other neurotic conditions that spring into being as the result of a trauma but which, since they are not differentiable from neuroses of nontraumatized individuals, are assumed by most psychiatrists to be merely the overt expression of a disease process that has been present but latent; the patient seizes on the fact of the trauma as an excuse for regressive behavior. The compensation may be money: and doctors have seen many cases of patients who remain ill until their legal day in court is over and then speedily regain their health. The compensation is not necessarily money: it may be the opportunity to avoid an unpleasant or threatening situation or a chance to retire to a condition of comparative invalidism for the attention and sympathy that can be gained.

Malingering is the conscious simulation of or stressing of illness in order to evade work or responsibility or to gain something else.

Dr. W. Donald Ross differentiated *traumatic neurosis* from *compensation neurosis* and *malingering* and stated that the traumatic neurosis definitely dates from the time of an injury or threat of injury, that the patient shows increased irritability and a startle reaction, and that there are repetitive dreams of again being in the danger situation. The compensation neurosis may only appear to have had its inception at the time of injury. This may be an artifact, and the onset of the illness may have been at an earlier period; in either case, a previously existing personality pattern is a contributing cause of the illness. The compensation neurosis does not have such clear-cut symptoms as increased irritability and the startle reaction and there is an absence of repetitive dreams. Said Dr. Ross:

I suggest that for "Traumatic Neurosis," the *causa sine qua non*, or the specific cause for each particular syndrome, is overwhelming psychic trauma or threat. Whereas, for "Compensation Neurosis," the particular cause, without which it would not be this particular syndrome, is the possibility of some monetary gain, or some other emotional gain from the persistence of symptoms.

To add to the complications of this comparison, however, an "unresolved traumatic neurosis" may be a factor precipitating the "compensation neurosis." "When the case is diagnosed as 'Traumatic Neurosis' only because of having been apparently precipitated by an injury, there may or may not have been an actual traumatic neurosis produced at that time. However, if a traumatic neurosis has remained unresolved, if it has not progressed with spontaneous recovery, or if there has not been appropriate treatment, then this individual, whatever his previous personality pattern, is more disposed to the regression and seeking of secondary gain which maintains the compensation neurosis."

Dr. Ross finds the presence of repetitive dreams a pathognomonic sign of the presence of a traumatic rather than some other type of psychoneurosis, and if the history of repetitive dreams cannot be elicited, "I have considerable question as to whether or not it is traumatic neurosis." Dr. Franz Alexander agreed that "repetitive dreams are most characteristic for a genuine traumatic neurosis. It is the expression of the ego's attempt of *postsequent* mastery of a traumatic situation." Dr. Herbert Modlin agreed that repetitive dreams were "almost pathognomonic of the condition."

But Dr. Gene Usdin, moderator, raised the question whether repetitive dreams—the outstanding diagnostic characteristic of the disease—really were "a *causa sine qua non* for the diagnosis of traumatic neurosis . . . it might seem that there are some other mechanisms that the ego could use instead of repetitive dreams." And Dr. Henry Brosin also challenged the essentiality of the repetitive dream criterion:

Apparently the essential criterion here is the presence of the repetitive dream. If we accept this criterion there is no need for further argument. However, we should be aware that not all definitions have included this criterion, and that consequently we are playing a kind of game. It is a serious game, to be sure. . . . In the future, we probably will have to arrive at several different levels of conceptualizations of the criteria of a traumatic neurosis as a psychological process, and not refer to this group of disorders as if they were an established entity about which there was no disagreement.

Dr. Brosin concluded that trauma is general and we are all victims of the disease. "In a special and limited sense our most useful clinical definition of traumatic neurosis is well known to us from everyday living. At one level of generalization above the clinical entity, 'trauma' is a commonplace event. We are constantly dealing with intrusions and discomforts in one way or another. In this sense we are all victims of a petit traumatic neurosis, hour by hour, as long as we live." And Dr. Alexander pointed out that he agreed with Freud that "every neurosis is a traumatic neurosis," the trauma being real or fantasied, a sexual assault, the loss of an important figure in life on whom one relies, losing a job, losing hope, as well as the more obvious physical trauma—such as an explosion—that is usually associated with traumatic neurosis.

The consensus of the Round Table appears to have been that traumatic neurosis is a diagnostic category distinct from other neurotic conditions, and that the diagnosis presupposes a mentally healthy individual who would not have developed the illness had it not been for a major trauma. In addition, some—but not all—of the participants saw the symptom of repetitive dreams in which the traumatic situation was relived as an essential or near-essential factor in arriving at the diagnosis. But in spite of the almost unanimity, the vexing question was raised whether this condition is necessarily related to external trauma—whether it is distinguishable from other cases of "breakdown" after a variety of life experiences, such as the death of a close relative.

If we go along with the majority and assume that there is a clearly defined psychiatric entity, which we will call *traumatic neurosis*, we have the problem of deciding whether the patient who acquires this condition should be compensated in a damage case, or in a case involving workmen's compensation or veteran's disability, in the same way that he would be compensated if a more clearly physical injury had been received. The decision is complicated by the fact that such authors as Smith and Solomon[30] and more recently Thompson[31] use the term *traumatic neurosis* differently from Ross, Usdin and other writers on the topic.

But we can clarify the situation by dealing with the cases in the three categories: *1.* traumatic neurosis—a healthy individual became mentally ill as the result of an overwhelming stress; *2.* compensation or triggered neurosis—the individual had a latent illness triggered or precipitated by the trauma and held onto by the patient for largely unconscious reasons; and *3.* malingering—the individual consciously deceives.

Thompson presumably would not object to this classification, since he stresses that many of the 500 litigated cases that he studied involved patients with preexisting neurotic traits of character; in fact, 87% in his series showed this predisposition to illness, in contrast to only 12% of a matched series of neurologic cases that showed preexisting neurotic tendencies. Many of the 87% would fall into the category of compensation neurosis, the test possibly being whether the traumatic stimulus that precipitated the neurosis would have had a similar effect, or might reasonably have had a similar effect, on a mentally healthy person.

Smith and Solomon similarly have divided the cases they studied—all of traumatic neurosis that reached appeals courts in Great Britain or the United States—into those where the stimulus was such that it *might* have sufficed to cause a neurosis in an average person and those where the stimulus did not appear to them to have been sufficient to cause a neurosis in the average person; and they too can be considered to follow roughly the more modern classification of traumatic and triggered neurosis. (Of 129 cases in which appeals courts upheld a verdict, they found only 13 where they believed an average person might have become neurotic—including the colorful example they list as A9: "A 165 pound chimpanzee entered plaintiff's house and in her presence attacked her two little children in succession, choking one of them severely and threatening plaintiff as well; plaintiff developed hysteria.")

Using the grouping, then, of traumatic neurosis, compensation neurosis and malingering, the question remains of compensation for the conditions. Or should the prevailing view be that which the Supreme Court of the State of Washington expressed a half century ago: "An allowance of damages in the cases of traumatic neurasthenia touches the border of speculation at best"?[32]

The pattern in these cases is that the courts are often dubious concerning the reality of the symptoms that the plaintiffs allege. Says Thompson: "Often, it is difficult to convince any tribunal that subjective symptoms are real. The presence of even a small amount of objective evidence will help." But once the court is willing to concede that a medical condition does exist, and that it has as its proximate cause the defendant's act or omission, then the compensation awarded will often be great. Psychiatrists may say that there is a difference between traumatic and compensation neurosis, but some courts appear to consider only the fact that a medical disease developed as a result of defendant's act or omission, and the defendant must pay the consequences.

The logic behind this view has often been expressed in the dictum that a tortfeasor takes his victim as he finds him. Say Smith and Solomon: "Both British and American courts, with a singular unanimity, have held that once a defendant can be culpably connected with the general type of injury he has caused the plaintiff to suffer, the bars are down. The defendant cannot then be heard to say: 'I should not be held to pay for the full harm but only for the degree of injury which a normally constituted person would suffer.'" An analogy is found in criminal law where a burglar who intends to rob but does not intend to kill is held for first degree murder if he accidently kills during the commission of the crime. So a negligent tortfeasor is held for all the consequences that result from his tort; we have already quoted Justice Kennedy in *Dulieu* vs *White and Sons* to the effect that "if a man is negligently run over or otherwise negligently injured, it is no answer to the sufferer's claim for damages that he would have suffered less injury, or no injury at all, if he had not had an unusually thin skull or an unusually weak heart."

Following this line of reasoning, some courts have said that if a plaintiff develops a neurosis following a tort, the tortfeasor cannot assert that the plaintiff had a predisposition or a tendency to have the neurosis. These courts, then, do not differentiate between traumatic and compensation neurosis. Some courts have gone so far as to rule that even though the secondary gain, the possibility of damages to be awarded as a result of the current litigation, has been a factor in the continuation of the neurosis, since the factor is largely unconscious and a part of the disease itself the defendant is not relieved of any liability by virtue of this circumstance. Moreover, although many psychiatrists feel that neuroses are not necessarily irreversible or permanently disabling, courts have often been persuaded by testimony that they are.

What all this means is that although courts tend to be reluctant to grant damages for traumatic or compensation neuroses, once the reluctance is overcome they will grant large damages and will disregard factors that seem important to the psychiatrist—such as the possible distinction between traumatic and compensation neurosis, the fact that the plaintiff may have had a history of previous emotional problems, and the fact that the disability the plaintiff claims is complete and permanent may not be so.

Solomon and Smith in their 1943 article (described by Curran[33] as "still the best article on the subject in the law reviews, and, I suspect, anywhere else") advocated an approach to the problem that permitted more gradations.

It is necessary in our opinion to take into account the pretraumatic personality for the purpose of discovering what part of the total injury really represents a preexisting neurotic constitution merely expressing itself by more obvious symptoms in response to stimuli which would cause no such symptoms in a normally constituted person. The legal import of this concept is enormous. It means that persons who develop more patent forms of neurosis in response to traumatic stimuli inadequate to so injure a normal person, are not caused thereby to develop the neurosis as a new and original condition. It is legally erroneous and socially unjust to compensate them on any such theory. Such cases are properly to be regarded as instances of aggravation of preexisting injuries or impairments, and so compensated modestly. The neurotic constitution is the major factor in the disability and it antedates the particular exacerbation of symptoms for which the plaintiff seeks damages.

These authors feel that remoteness of the expectation of the injury should run both to culpability and compensation. They believe that in cases without physical injury and where the psychic stimulus is slight (which outnumber major psychic stimulus cases by a ratio of 9:1 in their list of 129 cases where the appeals court sustained the award of damages), courts should find some way to deny recovery to the plaintiff. The court can rule that the causation is not truly proximate; or, failing this, that the result of the tort was too remote in expectation, so the actor was not really derelict in his duty; or, failing that, as a matter of judicial policy rule against the plaintiff on such grounds as difficulty of proof and judicial aversion to making the load of liability inordinately heavy. "We may hope and expect to see fuller and more effective use made of this doctrine of remoteness of damages."

But if all else fails—Smith and Solomon feel strongly on this subject—they wish courts to make new law to prevent neurotics from receiving possibly unjust deserts.

A bold court would be warranted in holding that the development of neurosis following a *minimal stimulus* or slight impact is an idiosyncratic response, in which cause-effect relationships are hopelessly obscured, and that difficulties of proof, appraisal and just compensation are so great as to raise an extrinsic policy against their redress. . . .

Even if courts are not willing to go this far to deny recovery, Smith and Solomon have another strategem up their legal sleeves.

Courts timid about thus cutting off entirely the liability for neurosis caused by stimuli too insubstantial and inadequate to so injure the average person, may limit the measure of damages by resorting to another principle. It is the rule everywhere that a plaintiff with a preexisting illness or impairment, cannot hold one who injures him liable in damages for his prior condition, but only for its aggravation. It is good logic and the better legal view that a defendant shall not be held liable for an injury, or any part thereof, which he did not cause if it is practicable to make a separation.

They feel that lack of proper information causes juries and courts to allow extravagant awards when plaintiffs have had idiosyncratic responses to minimal stimuli.

This disturbing phenomenon would soon be corrected if triers of fact and appeal judges realized that the neurotic who presents a deplorable spectacle in court was not immediately before the accident truly 'as fit as a fiddle' or 'the strongest woman in the house' or 'the picture of health.' A plaintiff can always bring trusting neighbors to court bearing witness to his hale and hearty pre-accident health, and ready to describe calamitous changes noticed in him shortly after receipt of the trivial impact. These laymen see only the flowering stalk of the neurosis, not the extensive roots underground, nor how the trivial stimulus, like a little rain water, combines with the sun's warmth and other environmental factors, to cause rapid surface growth. Actually, as we shall continue to stress, the trivial stimulus which causes appearance of new symptoms (or the flowering stalk of the neurosis) merely adds to a process already underway.

If we may shift metaphors, another fit analogy is to compare the waxing of this type of traumatic neurosis to the breaking open of an old scar, which has healed, only to break open at a later date in response to some trivial stress or some purposeful need of the individual.

Still again, we may compare the pretraumatic condition of such a neurotic to a cracked vase. The unobservant or untrained eye may not notice the crack, but only that the vase will hold water. It is only when the crack spreads and the vase will no longer hold water that he is conscious of any defect. But the law of torts must follow the rule of the market place and take cognizance that a cracked vase is not so valuable as an intact one. If the defendant's conduct causes the crack to spread, he may justly insist that he shall not make compensation on any assumption that the vase was previously perfect. So here, traumatic neurosis resulting from trivial stimuli should be treated as mere accession to, or aggravation of, a preexisting impairment. Once this truth is grasped we can expect to see the measure of damages lowered to more modest levels.

After describing a case in which the plaintiff was "permanently" disabled as a result of the traumatic neurosis, but shortly after receiving a $40,000 compromise settlement was able to resume her career as a concert singer, Smith and Solomon state:

The patient is never as badly off as he appears, the symptoms often lend themselves to dramatic presentation in court, the trier of fact is apt to gain the false impression that the plaintiff has sustained a calamitous permanent disability, and the injury is entirely ascribable to the defendant's fault. It demonstrates how the stresses, strains and excitement of litigation exacerbate symptoms, causing them on trial to appear more severe than they are. It shows, also, how rapid and unexpected may be the complete cure derived from a 'green-back plaster' in the form of a compromise settlement. . . .

They conclude that they "would be the first to proclaim" the reality of the traumatic neurosis, but they argue that this is a unique situation in the law of torts and the "naive all-or-none theory of causation" should not be the basis for the award of damages. In particular, they feel courts labor under a misapprehension concerning the permanence of neurotic disability. With this, they end their plea for smaller damages in the typical case of traumatic neurosis, characterized by both a stimulus that is less than overwhelming and a response to this stimulus that is idiosyncratic.

Siegal shares this view that awards are excessive in these cases.[34]

Due to the mistaken concept that traumatic neuroses involve permanent disability, courts have awarded excessive and unjust compensation. Many medical witnesses aid in this misapprehension by testifying carelessly that the condition is of uncertain or indefinite duration, and by such testimony the expert lays a false foundation for a judicial inference that the disorder is indeterminate in nature.

More recently Usdin[35] has also stressed the precarious balance of many of the plaintiffs in compensation neurosis cases before the trauma and urged a sharper differentiation by lawyers and psychiatrists of traumatic and compensation neuroses.

Thompson[36] and Watson[37] apparently take the opposite view, that courts should be readier to accept the contention of the plaintiffs that his subjective symptoms are real and worthy of compensation. In considering the following quotation from Thompson, one should keep in mind that he does not set up the separate classification of traumatic and compensation neuroses but lumps both groups together under the heading of posttraumatic psychoneurosis. He says that probably the best aid in convincing a tribunal that subjective symptoms are real "is the ability to demonstrate that posttraumatic psychoneurotic symptoms are part of a clearly defined syndrome, that they are not vague or intangible. A cross-examining attorney asked recently: 'Doctor, isn't the term "traumatic neurosis" a sort of a catchall or waste basket?' When it is pointed out to this attorney that a posttraumatic psychoneurosis is as distinct as a fractured femur, he may be willing to concede the point." Dr. Watson similarly feels that the ends of justice will be best served by a less strict differentiation of traumatic and compensation neurosis.

It is my impression that we will confuse the resolution of present legal situations if we go into court with . . . a narrow definition of traumatic neurosis. . . .
While indeed we may set up arbitrarily such a class of emotional illnesses, this
will be seriously confusing in the courtroom since it touches upon a point of
legal (*not* medical) policy, and without making this fact clearly apparent.

With psychiatric opinion ranged on both sides of the question of
more ready recovery in the compensation neurosis cases, no reputable
authority has appeared for the malingerer, who consciously deceives.
Many dynamic psychiatrists would probably argue that the malingerer,
who consciously knows that he is deceitful, is motivated to pursue his
deception by unconscious factors; the same line of reasoning would
hold that all criminals are psychiatrically ill, whether their crimes are
rational or irrational. The pragmatic argument against these extremist
opinions is that the structure of our legally based society would break
down if psychiatrists marked out as their area the totality of the conditions that present themselves to the court, leaving no ground for the
lawyer. Although some knowledge of the unconscious factors that
motivate the malingerer may add to understanding and even com-
passion, this still seems to be an area where both psychiatrist and
lawyer would find no basis for compensation.

Our conclusion has been that the law concerning mental suffering
and traumatic neuroses is still in the process of development, and
although the tendency has been to expand the area where awards will
be granted for mental suffering, there is no agreement on the subject
of traumatic neuroses. One exception must be noted. In workmen's
compensation cases, the law has been increasingly liberal in granting
recovery for compensation or triggered neurosis or even psychosis, in
spite of the fact that most psychiatrists would testify that the roots of
psychosis go deeply into the childhood history and possibly even into
the constitutional endowment of the individual, and that the connection between the psychic stimulus and the psychosis would be hard
to prove.

The workmen's compensation laws were set up as a type of industrial insurance, and the courts have felt that the standards that apply
in cases under these acts are not the same as those in tort cases. Bohlen
and Polikoff have given some of the reasons for the greater liberality
of courts in these cases.

Since the purpose of the Act is to give compensation for all such injuries as in
fact result from a work-accident, the liability may well extend further than
where it is imposed as a penalty for moral or social delinquency. Furthermore,
the fact that such cases are not tried by a jury, but by referees whose business
it is to constantly hear such cases, affords some protection against the danger
of fraud or exaggeration.[38]

Even though the initial proceeding in these cases is before a referee, the appeal is to a court, and once the case has been decided, it becomes a precedent citable when future cases come to trial. Almost inevitably, some of the decisions in the workmen's compensation cases will be felt in tort cases, because some courts will fail to differentiate the two types of cases and will assume that dubious causal connections of trauma and disease approved by a referee and upheld by an appellate court under the liberal workmen's compensation doctrine also apply to the same trauma and disease as they appear in a tort case. The basic difference is that in workmen's compensation cases an employer knows when he hires an employee that "he takes him as he finds him"—asthma, emphysema, hypertension, neurosis, or psychosis notwithstanding—and if the employee is injured or becomes ill it is the employer's responsibility. Whether this is good public policy—because it could encourage employers to hire only the young and the healthy, and it also gives the employer the right to invade the privacy of the potential employee by insisting on probing medical and psychiatric examinations—can hardly be raised at this late date. The facts are that the employer takes the employee with all his preexisting problems, and that the referees view these cases as insurance decisions rather than as assessments of blame.

Workmen's compensation case referees have been liberal in connecting not only a cause, sometimes apparently remote, and a disease, but also an incident that befalls an employee and the job he holds; "work-connected" has acquired a meaning that would seem broad to those who introduced this type of legislation a half century ago. The purpose of such legislation was to protect injured employees, who were under legal handicaps in seeking damages: they could not finance cases so easily as their employers, often had trouble persuading their fellows to testify in their behalf, and often lost their jobs because of the bad blood engendered by going to court at all. In addition, legal doctrines that had evolved concerning assumption of risk (the employee had "voluntarily" taken a job in a dangerous industry) and contributory negligency, by the employee himself or a fellow employee, often led to no recovery for the injury.[39] In spite of these difficulties in gaining redress, courts were burdened with negligence cases: "When the century opened most cases tried by civil courts of general jurisdiction were suits of injured workmen against their masters."[40] One of the purposes of the new legislation was to eliminate the concept of negligence from this type of suit and to make this an insurance matter rather than a tort case.

Whether the drafters of the legislation could have anticipated some recent decisions under workmen's compensation laws is doubtful. The *Wall Street Journal* reports,[41] in an article on the rising costs of job-linked ills, that "a California bank executive, visiting New York on a business trip, died in a fire in a hotel room with a female companion who wasn't his wife. Ultimately, the courts ruled that his widow was eligible for workmen's compensation benefits." The article continues, "An insurance man, recalling this case and a similar one involving a game warden, remarks scathingly, 'We're no longer surprised when benefits are awarded for injuries sustained while committing adultery'."

In one case, a 56-year-old employee who suffered a stroke while asleep in bed was awarded compensation on the evidence of his doctor, who attributed the stroke to overwork.[42] In another, the widow of a law-school dean submitted a claim after her husband died of a coronary occlusion while giving a speech to a legal fraternity. The state industrial commission rejected her contention that the heart attack was caused by law-school duties, but a district court, accepting testimony of a connection between the two, overruled the commission and awarded compensation.[43]

Courts have also stressed the fact that when referees find evidence, no matter how slight, to connect cause and effect, the appeals court does not have the right—unless the referees have no basis in the record for their findings—to challenge it. The appeals court is not a trier of fact but an arbiter of law.

The result of liberalized standards by referees and unwillingness of the appeals courts to rule on matters of fact has been felt in the area of workmen's compensation cases dealing with mental illness. Few cases of this kind were brought before 1940; they are now much more frequent.

Brill and Glass[44] describe three workmen's compensation cases in which mental or nervous disorders were attributed to emotional or psychic stress in the absence of physical injury or impact.

One of the early cases of this type involved a claimant who was frightened by an electric flash near her caused by a short circuit in a motor. She fainted and was caught before she fell by another employee. As a result of the mental association this created she fainted again the next time she saw this co-worker, and it became impossible for her to work because of this neurosis (*Burlington Mills* vs *Hagood*, 177 Va 204, 13 SE 2d 291, 1941).

A similar case in which compensation was awarded involved a claimant who developed a hysterical paralysis of her left side "as a result of" fright caused by a loud noise and flash of light created when lightning struck the building in which she worked. (*Charon's Case*, 321 Mass. 694, 75 NE 2d 511, 1947.)

These and other cases were the precedents on which current policies of many jurisdictions are based. Several states, notably New York, Indiana, New Jersey and Nebraska, still do not allow recovery for mental illness in the absence of some element of accidental physical injury. In Florida, if both the cause and the result are considered "mental," compensation will be denied under its statute which states that nervous or mental injury resulting from fright or excitement does not constitute compensable accidental injury.

The third and most important case is *Carter* vs *General Motors*,[45] where a precedent was established "of compensating an employee for a psychiatric breakdown not associated with any physical injury, accident, specific event, or unusual stress or incident." James Carter, a machine operator, developed paranoid schizophrenia, which he attributed to emotional pressure encountered on his job. He was an assembly line worker who—like the character portrayed by Charlie Chaplin in *Modern Times*—found the assembly line too fast and himself falling further and further behind in his job of filing and grinding hub assemblies. When he tried to compensate for his lag by taking hub assemblies to his work bench two at a time, he was reprimanded by his foreman on the ground that the assembly parts later became mixed on the conveyor belt. The "double bind" which has been described as part of the etiology of schizophrenia is apparent in the situation. "When he took only one hub assembly at a time he fell behind, and when he fell behind he would take two assemblies at a time, get them mixed up, and receive criticism from his foreman." He then suffered an emotional collapse, diagnosed as a paranoid schizophrenic reaction. Nine months later, after hospitalization, he filed a claim for compensation for permanent total disability, which the referees granted. The Supreme Court of Michigan, on an appeal by General Motors in 1960, decided that the disability was not permanent, but it did create forensic psychiatric history by affirming the award of damages for temporary disability. The court was aware that Carter's physician felt that he had had the predisposition towards the psychotic break for a number of years, but, since the causal chain of job-pressure and the outbreak of illness seemed complete, the compensation was granted.

The decision was not universally applauded. Said a dissenting Justice: "I do not believe that the injury arose out of employment. . . . there is nothing in this case identifiable as an occupational risk. The job was a simple job and the foreman's instructions were even more simple. Nothing more emanated from the employment. The disability arose out of the plaintiff's own feelings and misapprehension and from within himself completely." And Brill and Glass comment:

Life is characterized by stress, both interpersonal and intrapsychic. No job is free from stress. It is one thing to provide sickness insurance that will cover the varied manifestations of disordered emotional states, and it is another to attribute these states incorrectly to isolated or specific job stresses. There are two questions that society must answer: Who should be liable for the costs of mental disorders not expressly a result of work-related injury? To what extent are mental disorders caused by work?

Following the logic of *Carter* vs *General Motors*, all mental illness, neurotic and psychotic, incurred by an employee can be attributed to job pressure because there is always a history of increasing tensions on the job before any precipitate outbreak of mental pathology.

Nonlawyers understand that law is based on precedent, but they do not understand the efficient and complicated series of references and cross-references, based on coded key numbers, which enable a finding of one court to appear in another finding of the same or another court with amazing speed and ease. The findings in the Carter case were thus reduced to various numbered headings under the general topic of Workmen's Compensation and are available to all legal researchers hunting for precedents for such propositions as—

Workmen's Compensation 546. Where expert medical testimony indicated that machine operator had a personality disorder and a predisposition to development of a schizophrenic process, and operator suffered a disabling psychosis caused by emotional pressures produced by production line employment, he sustained a disability compensable under part 2 of the Workmen's Compensation Act.

Workmen's Compensation 517. It is not necessary to find an accident or a fortuitous event in order to grant an award under part 2 of the Workmen's Compensation Act.

The Carter case accordingly has been cited in an even more extreme case, which also arose under Michigan's Workmen's Compensation Law. The Supreme Court of Michigan stated in *Trombley* vs *Michigan*:

We have held that compensation benefits are payable for incapacity to work because of a claimant's mental disorder arising out of and in the course of his employment, whether or not such mental disorder results from a direct physical blow to claimant's body. *Carter* vs *General Motors Corporation*, 361 Mich. 577, at p. 585 and pp. 590–592, 106 N. W. 2d 105, and cases referred to therein. However, we have not had occasion previously to decide under what circumstances, if ever, death benefits are payable under our act if such work-connected mental disorder induces its victim to commit suicide. This case squarely presents that issue for decision.[46]

Trombley had been an attendant-nurse in a cottage at a Michigan home for mentally retarded persons. He was 37 years old, had served in the Army in World War II, and was hospitalized for asthma and neurosis, for which he received a disability pension of $100 a month. A patient in the cottage died, as a result of injuries, and the state legislature ordered an investigation, which was accompanied by newspaper, radio and television publicity. Trombley was one of the employees questioned on several occasions. The appeal board of the workmen's compensation commission found that the investigation precipitated a "drastic personality change in Trombley and produced in him mental depression so noticeable that it caused concern to those around him."

It found further that his suicide during the course of the investigation "was an uncontrollable impulse, not a voluntary action, and that it was caused directly by the investigations." An award of compensation to the widow was affirmed by the workmen's compensation commission appeal board. The Supreme Court of Michigan, by an evenly divided court, sustained the award of death benefits to the widow on the ground that the suicide was induced by work-connected mental disorder.

Brill and Glass think a possible rationale for the *Carter* case is that a worker who does not have health insurance and does not have substantial savings will have to be provided for either by workmen's compensation funds or by the community.

But the reasoning behind the determinations in workmen's compensations are often obscure, and a search of precedents finds contrary determinations on somewhat similar facts. In a Minnesota case, the suicide of a workman who had injured his back unloading pipe, had unsuccessful surgery for relief of pain and thereafter had domestic difficulties that culminated in his suicide, more than three years after the original injury was held to be not work-connected. And in the cases involving nonpsychiatric conditions, one court will find that tenosynovitis resulted from use of a calculating machine, while another court will hold that headaches that require hospitalization in an employee with high blood pressure were not connected with the exertion of climbing a ladder at work.

In spite of some laggard jurisdictions, the tendency for referees and courts to extend the area in which claims will be recognized under the workmen's compensation laws has its repercussions in other fields of law dealing with recovery for psychiatric illness. Cases involving mental pain and suffering and neurosis—even when the neurosis is stipulated to be a compensation neurosis, where the possibility of a legal award is a factor in the perpetuation of the neurosis—reflect the inflationary trends towards a broader scope for the finding of responsibility and a higher determination of the amount of damages.

CHAPTER 13

Admissions, Commitment and Committability

WHEN a competent patient enters an ordinary hospital, he enters into a contract, express or implied, with the hospital. The hospital contracts to give him proper care during his stay; he contracts to abide by the rules of the hospital and to pay his bill.

During his stay in the hospital, he may become violent. He may become toxic, as a result of the disease or the treatment, and develop a psychosis; he may become uncontrollable after anesthesia. The hospital has the obligation and the right so to control him that he does not harm himself or others. If a delirious postoperative patient were left unguarded by an open window and jumped from it, the hospital would be considered negligent; and the hospital can forcibly restrain such a patient.[1]

But the right to restrain a patient is only a right limited to the duration of real necessity. While no one would challenge the right of a hospital to use restraints to prevent a delirious patient from pulling out intravenous tubing or a catheter, in most situations a hospital cannot interfere with the actions of a patient. If he curses or shouts obscenities but does not present a threat to himself or others, a hospital cannot tie him down or lock him up, unless it wishes to risk the possibility of a suit for false imprisonment.

Prosser has defined false imprisonment (sometimes called false arrest) as "the confinement of the plaintiff within boundaries fixed by the defendant, without legal justification, by an act or the breach of a duty intended to result in such confinement," and he notes that the Restatement of Torts has taken the position (although the case law on the subject is scanty) that there cannot be false imprisonment unless the plaintiff is aware of it, arguing that the right is one of freedom to go where he pleases, and that until he is aware of restraint there is no interference with it. (Accordingly, locking up an unconscious person would probably not constitute false imprisonment, nor would the use of restraints to hold down a patient not aware that he was being restrained.) The restraint need not be physical; threats of force are sufficient. It may be brief and need not be injurious; says Prosser, "The imprisonment need not be for more than an appreciable length of time, and it is not necessary that any damage result from it, since the tort is complete with even a brief restraint of the plaintiff's freedom."[2]

In addition, one who is physically restrained may have an action for battery (an unconsented-to physical contact that need not be hostilely intended and does not necessarily inflict harm) or for assault (the placing in apprehension of battery without the requirement of actual contact, as when the defendant fires at but misses the plaintiff).[3]

In order to minimize the difference between mental illness and other forms of illness, to keep the patient from being stigmatized by a stay in a mental hospital, and to encourage patients to seek prompt treatment in their own communities if they are suffering from mental or emotional problems, the general hospital is increasingly being made the hospital of first resort. But general hospitals accept only voluntary patients, and for a patient to be admitted to a general hospital there should be an assumption—quite fictitious with the victim of a stroke or some other condition causing unconsciousness—that this is in accordance with the patient's wishes. If a patient actively opposes the hospitalization, he can be held only if he is a threat to himself or others and only for that period necessary to summon the police or arrange for some other disposition of the problem. Those who advocate the greater use of general hospital wards for psychiatric hospitalizations are sometimes unaware of the limited control that the general hospital can exercise over the patient without risk of lawsuit.

The problem of dealing with patients whose liberties have to be abridged, and who have to be subjected to procedures to which they are unwilling to give consent, has led to the establishment of a special class of hospitals subject to greater control by the state than the general hospital but also given more freedom to deal with patients. This freedom involves the right to impose on those patients specified by statute as appropriately belonging in such hospitals restraints and procedures that otherwise would be considered not only torturous but also tortious.

Who are the mentally ill who can be involuntarily hospitalized? The Draft Act, prepared by the National Institute of Mental Health as a proposed model mental health code, defines a mentally ill individual, using a somewhat circular definition, as "an individual having a psychiatric or other disease which substantially impairs his mental health."[4] A typical definition, found in the Idaho code, has two parts and includes both the concepts of need of the patient for hospitalization and/or the fact that his mental condition makes him a danger to himself or to others.[5] "Mentally ill person or individual shall mean a person or individual who comes under either or both of the following descriptions: *1*. who is in such mental condition that he is in need of supervision, care or restraint; *2*. who is of such mental condition that he is dangerous to himself or to the person or property of others and is in need of supervision, care or restraint." Some states, such as Alabama, define mental illness or insanity for purposes of eligibility for psychiatric hospitalization in terms of the judicial determination that such illness is present: "A person shall be adjudged insane who has been found by a proper court sufficiently deficient or defective mentally to require that, for his own or others' welfare, he be removed to the insane hospital for restraint, care and treatment."[6]

Deutsch has pointed out that, during the Colonial period, the only laws concerning the violent and dangerously insane dealt with detention under the authority of the sovereign's police powers.[7] A Massachusetts statute of 1676 ordered the selectmen of towns with "dangerously distracted persons" to take care of them "that they do not damnify others." No statutes specifically concerned hospitalization. From the time the first asylums for the mentally ill were established, in the mid-1700's, until the post-Civil War period, the commitment of patients under statutory authority to these hospitals was effected easily, often merely on the request of a friend or relative. The commitment could be a hastily scribbled few words on a scrap of paper signed by a member of the hospital staff. Mrs. E. P. W. Packard, who was released from the Illinois State Hospital in 1863 after spending three years there, wrote two books and gave numerous lectures on the conditions in that institution, and pointed out that under the Illinois commitment statute married women could be involuntarily committed, on the judgment of the medical superintendents of the state asylum at Jacksonville, "at the request of the husband . . . without the evidence required in other cases," if they were evidently insane or "distracted." Infants could be similarly committed at the request of their guardians without the presentation of evidence ordinarily required. Mrs. Packard's thesis was that her husband had used the commitment as a way of triumphing in a marital dispute. Largely due to her efforts, Illinois enacted the so-called personal liberty bill, which required a jury trial to determine if commitment was appropriate.

Comments the American Bar Foundation's Report[8]:

Crusades by Mrs. E. P. W. Packard, Dorothea Dix, and others spurred the enactment of commitment laws which specified the use of judicial procedures designed to guard against wrongful commitments. The success of these earlier crusades is reflected in the almost single-minded concern with the possibility of wrongful commitment which characterized the legislative approach to the problems of the mentally ill until very recently.

There is some evidence that the contemporary legislative approach is more comprehensive. During the last twenty years many state legislatures have evidenced more concern about the treatment and rehabilitation of the mentally ill than the problem of wrongful commitment. Moreover, the advances in psychiatric knowledge together with the greater understanding of the attributes of mental health have supplied legislators with the factual basis necessary for the enactment of that legislation most conducive to the effective treatment of persons who are, in fact, mentally disabled. Many of the new laws have incorporated measures advocated by the medical profession, e.g., hospitalization by medical certification, emergency procedures, and temporary or observational procedures. A number of these laws included provisions designed to modernize the terminology used in determining to whom and under what circumstances involuntary hospitalization statutes should be applied. These legislative changes have not been viewed with equal favor by all observers. The propriety, and indeed the constitutionality, of some of the newer hospitalization procedures have been challenged. What constitutes the proper criteria for hospitalization, for example, remains open to question. . . .

Of course, if a patient decides voluntarily to enter a psychiatric hospital, many of the problems dealing with the criteria for commitment do not arise. And so the voluntary admission of the psychiatric patient has been advocated as an answer to difficulties here. England has led the way by making voluntary admissions to its psychiatric hospitals the rule rather than the exception.

The Draft Act, the proposed model law to govern the hospitalization of the mentally ill prepared by the National Institute of Mental Health, provides for voluntary admissions, along with other types of admissions procedures, for a variety of reasons[9]:

Voluntary admissions reduce the harmful experiences associated with compulsory hospitalization.
The mentally ill and their families are encouraged to obtain care at an early stage, when the promise of recovery is greatest.
The voluntary patient is more likely to cooperate with his physician.

Making hospitalization more readily available to the mentally ill should reduce the financial and human cost of mental illness, which is greatest when the patient's condition has been aggravated by delay in treatment. State legislatures recognize the desirability of voluntary admission of the mentally ill; with the exception of Alabama, all states provide that patients may apply for their own admission. Despite all this, statistics compiled by the World Health Organization indicate that only 10% of psychiatric hospitalizations in the United States are on a voluntary basis,[10] as compared with 85% in England and Wales[11] and 67% in Scotland.[12]

Why is the voluntary admissions procedure less utilized than it might be? One reason is that it is not really voluntary in the same way that admission to a general hospital is voluntary. When a patient voluntarily signs himself into a mental hospital, almost universally he agrees that, if and when he decides to depart the hospital, he must notify the staff and at this point can be detained against his will for a specified period. It is easier to get into a psychiatric hospital voluntarily than to get out voluntarily.

The Application for Voluntary Admission used in Pennsylvania, for example, states: "Application is hereby made for voluntary admission under the provisions of Section 301, 302 and 304 of the Mental Health Act of 1951 as amended. . . . The undersigned understands that he must give at *least ten days' notice in writing* to the Superintendent if it is desired that the patient leave the hospital.[13]

If the patient gives his ten days' notice in writing, he need not be detained; the hospital can let him go immediately. But the hospital does have a period of ten days in which to determine if it is in the patient's best interest to leave the hospital; and if the hospital staff disagrees with the patient about the wisdom of the discharge, it will proceed during this period to have the patient seen by two physicians (almost invariably psychiatrists, although the law does not specify that the physicians must be specialists) and, if possible, committed. The patient who signs himself into a psychiatric hospital voluntarily may sometimes feel as if he has put his neck in a noose.

The Report of the American Bar Foundation gives some reasons why the voluntary admission procedure in most states has received "insufficient utilization":

It has been suggested that more people have failed to use the procedures for voluntary admission largely because of the general inadequacy of the statutes providing for hospitalization in this manner. It must be noted at the very beginning of this discussion that hospitalization for the treatment of mental illness, as distinguished from a physical illness, may affect the patient's civil rights. Under such circumstances it is reasonable to assume that a potential applicant, at least one who is in sufficient contact with reality, would desire precise information concerning his right to admission and discharge as well as the effect hospitalization would have on his legal competency. Similarly, his decision might be influenced by the effect such an admission would have on his freedom to correspond with friends, to have visitors, to drive an automobile, and to exercise fully certain other personal and civil rights. The percentage of those using the procedures for voluntary admission is much higher where there are statutes protecting these rights, and the possibility of early and successful treatment increases accordingly.

Another reason for the relatively small number of voluntary admissions may be the overcrowded conditions of many mental hospitals. In most states the decision to admit voluntary patients is left to the discretion of the hospital authorities, who may hesitate to accept additional patients if the hospital's facilities are already overtaxed. This situation becomes even more complicated in those states where it is mandatory, regardless of the space then available in the institution, that a patient be admitted when hospitalized by a court.

Finally, it may be suggested that such admissions are few in number because only a small percentage of the mentally ill either recognize their own mental condition or are capable of initiating positive action on the basis of their knowledge.[14]

At least two other major problems remain to complicate the subject of voluntary admissions. We have talked, in our discussion of major legal themes that run through all branches of law, about contractual ability, which depends on sufficient ability to think and to understand so that the two parties entering into a contractual relationship—herewith, the voluntary patient and the hospital or its superintendent—have a "meeting of the minds" regarding the terms of the contract. Patients who are grossly disturbed (that is, psychotic), senile, or semicomatose do not have the ability to enter into a binding agreement. Many patients who need hospitalization cannot or should not seek it voluntarily because of a lack of contractual ability. The question arises, too, whether juveniles, who have limited ability at law to enter into contracts on their own behalf, can sign themselves into a hospital voluntarily; hospitals in some jurisdictions require both the juvenile and his parent (or guardian) to sign the voluntary admission application, but it is questionable whether the additional signature of an adult legalizes a contractual agreement that would be dubious otherwise.

In one state, Pennsylvania, a special provision of the statute designed to protect juveniles who become voluntary patients has resulted in the policy of some hospitals of refusing to admit juveniles on a voluntary basis. In Pennsylvania, few admissions to mental hospitals are by court order; a modern mental health code provides alternate methods of involuntary commitment that are less cumbersome and time-consuming. However, juveniles who enter hospitals voluntarily, after thirty days automatically become the subject of a court proceeding. "Under no circumstances, shall a person under twenty-one years of age, admitted voluntarily, remain a patient for more than thirty days unless prior to the expiration of such thirty day period an order of court is obtained committing the person to the institution. It shall be the duty of the Department of Public Welfare to advise the person admitted of his right to release unless such order of court is obtained and also of his rights with respect to the hearing before the court."[15] Rather than subject themselves to the time-consuming court hearing, some hospital administrators have arbitrarily decided not to admit juveniles on a voluntary basis.[16]

Even more complicated from a legal point of view is that in some jurisdictions statutes provide that the fact of mental hospitalization alone is sufficient to establish legal incompetency. Although voluntary admissions are allowed in some of these states, a patient who voluntarily enters a hospital and is thereupon presumed to be incompetent would find himself in a tenuous position if he then decides he does not want to be in the hospital. Only a handful of states—Illinois, New York, Ohio, Oklahoma, Tennessee, Texas and Wyoming—have statutes that expressly provide that voluntary patients retain their competency. Three other states, which do not deal with this specific question, do have statutory provisions regarding involuntary patients, specifying that these are not incompetent specifically as the result of hospitalization; so in these states—Arizona, Delaware and South Dakota—by analogy it would seem that voluntary patients would not be considered incompetent.[17]

Informal admission is a type of voluntary admission with a minimum of formality in signing papers and with the patient retaining the right to depart the hospital whenever he wishes. Modeled on the English practice, this type of admission has been adopted recently by four states: Connecticut, Illinois, Massachusetts and New York. Patients retain all rights, including the right to vote.[18] Use of this type of admission answers the objections of defenders of civil rights, who object to the voluntary admissions procedure found in other jurisdictions—voluntary about entering but not about leaving the hospital, and involving loss or possible loss of civil liberties. But because informal admission gives the hospital no handle by which to grab the patient—he can refuse any treatment and can leave whenever he wishes—hospital administrators and psychiatrists are reluctant to hospitalize most patients by such a procedure. Since a characteristic of mentally ill patients is an inability to recognize the need for treatment, many of these patients presumably would exercise their right to leave.

The Report of the American Bar Foundation makes three concise statements regarding the policy of voluntary admissions.[19] The use of voluntary admission procedure should be encouraged; the confusion surrounding the legal status of voluntary patients discourages the use of this procedure; voluntary patients should be entitled to and advised of the right to be released.

INVOLUNTARY COMMITMENT PROCEDURES

For the majority of mentally ill patients who will not enter hospitals on a voluntary basis, there are four main categories of involuntary commitment procedures—emergency, judicial, medical and observational.

EMERGENCY COMMITMENT

The application for admission for emergency care is usually a simplified form, effective in getting a patient into a hospital with a minimum of delay but valid only for a very limited duration of hospitalization. The patient's freedom is abridged but, since the abridgment is for a medical purpose and for only a limited time, it does not seem inappropriate under the circumstances. The American Bar Foundation's Report points out that the emergency care commitment is not really a hospitalization procedure but rather a form of detention; "unlike hospitalization, which undertakes to provide relatively permanent measures for the personal safety, treatment, and care of the mentally ill, detention has only limited short-range goals. It is concerned with the suppression and prevention of conduct likely to create a 'clear and present danger' to persons or property. Under common law, any official or private person has the right to detain a dangerous mentally ill person. The majority of jurisdictions have special statutory provisions for the emergency detention of the mentally ill. Thirteen states, however, lack such provisions."[20]

Of 36 jurisdictions that name in their statutes appropriate places for the emergency detention of the mentally ill, 20 mention both public and private hospitals, 14 only public hospitals, one private hospitals only, and another merely provides "some suitable place."[21]

In large urban centers and regions near state mental hospitals, hospitals are the ordinary places of detention; in other areas the jail is often the place of detention.

The jail is apparently a permissible place of detention for the mentally ill in most states. A few states either specifically prohibit the detention of the mentally ill in jails or provide that this is to take place only if the jail has special facilities or permit such action only in cases of extreme emergency. Because of the lack of authority and funds for the establishment of facilities to replace the jail, these statutory prohibitions are frequently ineffective.[22]

If jail is allowed as a place of detention, some jurisdictions specify that the patient can be detained only a very limited time. Massachusetts, for example, which allows emergency detention for five days in a hospital, allows it for only twelve hours in a jail. In most jurisdictions, emergency detention—whether in jail or hospital—is for a maximum period, which ranges from 24 hours in Colorado and the District of Columbia to 30 days in Connecticut, Illinois, Louisiana, Oklahoma, South Carolina, and South Dakota. The period specified in most statutes is in the range of five to ten days. In some jurisdictions no specific number of days is provided; the detention is for the period until a psychiatric examination shall have been completed. Other jurisdictions with specified maximum times allow the patient to be further detained if legal proceedings for his continued hospitalization have been commenced.[23]

The application for emergency detention is made in some states by a relative or friend; in some by any reputable citizen; in some others only by attending physicians or law enforcement or health officers or other public officials. States with modern mental health codes often specify that the application should be in two parts, one part to be signed by a relative or friend (who in the absence of anyone closer in the case of a vagrant or an indigent might be a police officer or other not usually considered to be encompassed within the definition of "friend") and the other part to be signed by a physician (not necessarily a psychiatrist, although sometimes the criteria listed state that a psychiatrist need have been in practice for a shorter period of time than another physician making the application).

The emergency care is always for a limited time; at the end of that time it is not renewable, and if the patient is to be continued to be held, he must either sign himself into the hospital as a voluntary patient or be committed under a formal procedure. Although theoretically the emergency care procedure represents a special admission procedure designed to deal expeditiously with acute emergency situations, in actual practice it is often used as a normal admission procedure in cases where it seems easier to have a simple form filled out rather than to fill out and have notarized the more complex forms used in more formal admission procedures. If a patient admitted to the hospital under this procedure can stay in the hospital for 20 to 30 days or for an indeterminate period (the case in 18 jurisdictions), many hospitalizations will fall completely within this time span. Hospitals in time have relied on this "emergency admission procedure" as a normal commitment for short-term hospitalization or a normal "preliminary" admission for longer-term care, in spite of the fact that legislatures probably did not intend the temporary care procedure to be used for this purpose.

JUDICIAL COMMITMENT

Judicial hospitalization procedures have been most used during the past century. A procedure is classified as judicial when a judge or jury has discretion to determine on the merits whether hospitalization is required by the applicable statutory provision. After the era of informal hospitalization procedures and starting with the post-Civil War period, judicial hospitalization was paramount, and its formalities—including notice, public hearing, right to counsel, often trial by jury, the taking of a record subject to review by a superior court—were seen as safeguards to prevent the railroading of well people into psychiatric hospitals. Judicial hospitalization procedures are still provided for by statute in thirty-seven jurisdictions, but judicial hospitalization, in spite of all safeguards, has been falling into increasing disrepute for a variety of reasons. The public nature of a judicial hospitalization stigmatizes the patient, the details of his illness become a matter of record, and newspaper publicity often results. The trial aspect of the proceeding involves delay and expense, including the hiring of counsel.

An editorial, "On Committing the Mentally Ill," in the *Medical Annals of the District of Columbia*,[24] comments on the expense of committing the uncooperative patient. Although the law for the District was modernized in 1964, the situation described still exists in many other jurisdictions. The safeguards so that due process will be observed "are not only numerous but so cumbersome and costly as to interfere seriously with the prompt institution of proper treatment in many cases." The costs are enumerated. "Engaging an attorney to file a petition in court and to follow the case through to adjudication may cost anywhere from $100 to $300. The psychiatrist's services, which include examining the patient, writing a report, and testifying before the Commission on Mental Health, may be from $100 to $150. Under the third method (of commitment provided by statute), the medical fees for two physicians to examine the patient, complete the certificates, and testify before the Commission may be from $150 to $200. In addition, the guardian *ad litem* appointed by the court . . . is usually awarded $50 if the estate is solvent. Combined legal and medical fees may, therefore, run from $200 to $500 depending on which method of commitment is used."

The judicial commitment not only involves expense and delay; often the hearing itself is a formality that does not take the time to delve into the merits of the individual case. Dr. Thomas J. Scheff, University of Wisconsin sociologist, who studied the judicial commitment procedures of 20 counties of a midwestern state, reported that one psychiatrist spent an average of 9.2 minutes with each of eight patients he was examining for court purposes and that one court—the one with the most cases—averaged 1.6 minutes per commitment, sometimes cutting off the patient in the middle of a sentence.[25]

When the judicial determination has been made that hospitalization is necessary, in many jurisdictions the patient is thereby adjudged insane, with the resulting stigma and loss of civil rights. Although the court theoretically continues to watch over the welfare of the committed patient, in actual practice the overworked judiciary cannot follow the progress of all these cases. When the patient is recovered, or when even such a minor change in his status as permission to leave the hospital to visit his family is required, the court must be petitioned. Perhaps the most important of the objections to judicial hospitalization in those jurisdictions where there is a right to jury trial is that twelve jurors do not always seem to be the appropriate arbiters of technical matters of mental health. Another compelling argument against judicial commitment procedures is that disturbed mental patients are the least able of most classes of citizenry to see that their rights are preserved in a judicial proceeding, although the opposing argument—that one who does not have sufficient mentation to protect his legal rights probably needs hospital care—may also seem valid.

Most states with judicial hospitalization procedures also have some provisions for a prehearing medical (that is, psychiatric) examination, so that the courtroom battle of opposing experts can be minimized. Judicial hospitalization remains the most common method of hospitalizing the mentally ill, but administrative commitments and involuntary medical commitments are finding increasing use and favor.

Some jurisdictions employ an *administrative board* rather than a judge or jury to determine the need of hospitalization, and on the basis of its investigation and, possibly, hearing, hospitalization for an indeterminate period can be ordered. The board is usually composed wholly or largely of physicians. The Report of the American Bar Foundation states that advocates of this approach believe that it is more akin to the "scientific approach" than judicial commitment. But it adds that "the position of the advocates of administrative hospitalization fails to take into consideration the fact that the ultimate decision on hospitalization is a social decision, rather than a medical one. Physicians are no more qualified to balance individual liberty against the social policy of the state or its police powers than are other groups. In fact, physicians may be less qualified than such a group as the judiciary."[26]

MEDICAL COMMITMENT

Involuntary commitment by medical certification describes the procedure by which an individual may be hospitalized for an indeterminate period without his consent and over his objection on the basis of certificates of one or more physicians. This procedure is designed largely to replace the judicial or administrative commitment. In some cases, the approval or endorsement of a judge is necessary, but the function of the judge here is not to review the merits of the case or to determine if hospitalization is desirable, but merely to verify the genuineness of the certificates and the qualifications of the examining physicians. Eleven states provide for medical commitments.[27]

The committed patient does have a right to a judicial review of his medical certification or, alternatively, the right to be released after notice, but few of these states require that he be notified of these rights, and despite the flexibility and freedom from legal technicalities of this procedure, the question whether it meets constitutional standards of due process continues to be perplexing.

The Missouri case of *State* vs *Mullinax*[28] involved a statute that had incorporated Section 6 of the Draft Act, which provides for involuntary hospitalization on written application by various designated citizens, plus certification by two designated medical examiners that the patient is mentally ill and either likely to injure himself or others or needs care or treatment in a mental hospital. The court stated that in exercise of police powers, the state might thus temporarily detain an allegedly insane person dangerous to himself or to others, but that, in other cases, the lack of notice and of an opportunity to be heard before being hospitalized, and the placing of the burden of requesting release or judicial hearing on the individual (who might be unaware of his rights to these alternatives) did create a lack of due process. The Missouri act was amended after this decision to provide that notice of all emergency detentions be given to the Probate Court, which is to order release of the patient if a judicial proceeding is not initiated within five days. The medical commitment in this case becomes not a separate admissions procedure but a temporary procedure pending use of a judicial commitment order.

In a state using the medical commitment (Pennsylvania is used here as an example), the following technical requirements must be observed. All three parts of the application—the relative's and the two physicians'—must be signed and sworn to before a notary. The notary must be of that, not a neighboring, state. The relative or friend must be a United States citizen. He must state that he believes that the patient is mentally ill and that care in a mental hospital is necessary for his benefit, and give facts about his behavior to support this view. Each of the two physicians must have resided in the state for at least one year, be licensed to practice in the state, and in addition have had at least one year's mental hospital experience as a physician or been in the actual practice of medicine or osteopathy for three years; his conclusions must be based on direct examination of the patient—not second-hand or hearsay facts—and the admission of the patient to the hospital must occur within thirty days of the first examination. The physician, who need not be a psychiatrist, may not be related by blood or marriage either to the patient or to the individual making out the relative's part of the application. The requirements concerning residency and notarization are designed to make sure that the physicians are available during any subsequent judicial proceeding.[29]

Another type of medical certification, very different from that under discussion in its legal implications, is *the nonprotested admission*. Under this procedure, provided for by statute in 14 states, one or more physicians by certificate can hospitalize a patient for an indeterminate time but only if the patient does not protest the procedure. This procedure thus falls halfway between the voluntary and the medical commitments. Some of the statutes do not clearly spell out the form that the patient's consent should take or, alternatively, the steps that should be taken to inform him of his right to protest.[30]

OBSERVATIONAL AND OTHER COMMITMENT

Observational commitment resembles in 16 states medical and in 23 states judicial commitment, but it is designed only to help formulate a diagnosis or to determine whether longer-term commitment is required, and accordingly is for only a specified time. In the typical statute, that time is specified as 30, 40, 60 or 90 days, although the range is from seven days in New Jersey to six months in Georgia, Idaho, Michigan, Missouri, New Mexico, Utah and West Virginia.[31]

Finally, varieties of commitment procedures are provided by statute for certain categories of persons. Many states have special commitment laws for addicts or alcoholics, which take into consideration the fact that these patients may not fall within the general definition of the insane or obviously need hospital care to the untrained observor's eye. Such laws are treatment-oriented, and commitments usually are not for an indeterminate period of time but rather subject to renewal at such intervals as every six months or every year.

Like a commitment yet not a commitment is a type of observational detention often imposed on persons picked up by the police and accused of committing a crime. If the crime appears to be irrational, such as some sexual offense (particularly those involving molesting children), or crimes involving thefts without financial motivation, judges under the authority of appropriate statutes will often send the accused to a state hospital for a specified period in order that he may be studied and a report sent to the court. This category of commitment, which involves the denial of liberty to one accused of a crime but not convicted, and involves also an enforced doctor-patient relationship of an often unwilling patient and a doctor whose role is not therapeutic but investigatory and reportorial, and whose participation is at the will not of the patient but of the state, raises complicated issues both of civil rights and of the doctor-patient relationship. The extralegal and extra-ethical characteristics of these commitments usually go unchallenged since the accused, who often is guilty of the alleged offense and knows he is liable to a possible jail sentence, is not in a position to protest his detention without the risk of incurring judicial wrath.

CLASH OF PHILOSOPHIES

The conflict between the need to hold the mentally ill for treatment and the need to preserve liberties guaranteed by the Constitution has resulted in wide swings in policy concerning commitments. We are now at a point in history where one swing has gone so far that forces are mobilizing to counteract it. Originally, commitment was an informal procedure with little attention paid to safeguarding civil liberties; the signature of a hospital official saying that he had received the patient was often the only document in the case. During the Civil War period, attention began to be paid to the plight of inmates held against their wills in unspeakable institutions, and, in response to public feeling, legislatures passed commitment laws putting all manner of judicial safeguards into the procedure. This was the era of the judicial commitment and the high point of legalism.

Psychiatrists pointed out the inhumanity of these laws. A bewildered psychotic patient would be forced to appear in a public judicial proceeding, sometimes held for the duration of his court appearance in handcuffs or restraints. The public nature of the proceeding kept the mentally ill from seeking treatment. The delay in getting the sick patient into the hospital was harmful to treatment, and in the case of a suicidally depressed patient might be fatal. Gradually, a more humane type of commitment, in which the judicial process was bypassed, became popular; the doctor rather than the judge had the responsibility for the decision, although the court remained in the background as a last resort for those who felt that commitment was unjustified. The trend towards easier commitment in the last decade has resulted in comprehensive revisions of the laws of such populous states as Illinois, New York, Ohio, and Pennsylvania. The New York revised mental hygiene law, which went into effect in 1965, for example, gives physicians rather than judges the authority to determine when an individual should be hospitalized, with the courts, however, continuing to rule on the involuntary commitment of persons suspected of criminal acts who "do not act in the manner of a sane person." The new law outlaws indefinite hospitalization of noncriminal patients without legal review. A special agency, believed to be unique among the states, will see that patients have court hearings if they desire them; it will inform patients and relatives and other interested persons periodically concerning the patient's legal rights. In addition, the voluntary hospitalization procedure has been put on an informal basis, ensuring easy admission for nonprotesting patients, but this type of hospitalization is only for a specified time. The records of all patients will be reviewed by the court at intervals of six months, one year, and every two years thereafter.[32]

But modern and liberalized mental health laws have aroused the opposition of two groups particularly concerned with Constitutional safeguards—the politically conservative and the legally vigilant. Says Curran, "It is ironic that the mental health movement may find itself attacked on the left by the civil rights advocates and on the far right by the John Birch Society and its strange bedfellows."[33] Not all the opposition to liberalization of commitment procedures comes from the left and the far right, however, nor are all civil rights advocates political extremists.

In one jurisdiction, a recently enacted revision of the commitment laws tightened the court control of hospitalization procedures and hospitalized patients. The new District of Columbia law provides for emergency hospitalization of only 48 hours before a court order must be sought, and a "right to treatment" under which a patient can be released if he can show the court that he is receiving inadequate treatment; retains a review procedure before a Commission on Mental Health, and jury trials on commitment; and removes from the mental hospital the discretionary power in controlling voluntary admissions who wish to leave it.[34] Says Curran of the new District of Columbia law:[35]

Unlike the law in most states, it was not advocated by mental health professions or lay mental health organizations. It was the product of lawyers and others interested mainly in constitutional civil rights. Civil rights groups are becoming more and more interested in the commitment laws. They can be a serious obstacle to the efforts of mental health people to make treatment easier to obtain and communications between hospital and community freer and more open. . . . In some areas, these groups are, in my judgment, on sound grounds constitutionally and many of the provisions they support, such as periodic re-evaluation, are quite commendable.

Against the background of the clash of philosophies, some psychiatric voices are raised to question the usefulness of hospitals. A New York study indicates that day care for psychotics was as effective for treatment as a traditional in-patient service.[36] A professor of psychiatry protests that the mental patient is degraded by having commitment or treatment forced on him, under the contention that the patient does not know what is best for himself.

We ought to frankly recognize that psychiatric commitment is a form of social control and not a form of treatment for illness. The humanism of rule of law is based on procedural restraints on the arbitrary exercise of state power; it is only diluted if that power is smuggled in with a psychiatric disguise. If there is a social mandate for the control of certain types of behavior, let it be openly and frankly exercised under the scrutiny of an informed citizenry, rather than covertly as a medical practice.[37]

Despite some questioning of the effectiveness of the mental hospital and some advocacy of eliminating commitments, the procedure will be with us for a time and the controversy concerning legalistic versus liberal commitment laws will continue.

Whatever the type of commitment—voluntary with the right to hold the patient after he gives notice of his intention to leave, judicial, administrative, medical, nonprotested medical, observational, or detentional—inequities are inherent in a situation where the medical needs of the patient may be in conflict with his guaranteed freedoms. Inevitably, the doctor will stress the need for treatment and tend to be oblivious of the patient's civil liberties; equally inevitably, the lawyer and the judge will be more interested in the preservation of individual rights than in the necessity for enforced medical care.

Part of the problem is that the patient himself thinks of hospitalization as a punishment very like some criminal penalties, and the structure of the state hospital system in many jurisdictions—where little intensive treatment can be furnished to the average patient because of staff shortages and limitations of facilities—encourages the resistance to voluntary admission. But even with ideal hospital conditions, the mental patient will tend to minimize his need for treatment—that being part of his psychiatric problem—and the legislator, the court, and the physician will continue to have the difficult task of determining whether the patient's need for treatment or his right to liberty takes precedence and, where these two overlap, how and to what extent they can be reconciled.

CHAPTER 14

Rights of Hospitalized Patients

WHEN a competent patient is treated in an ordinary hospital, the civil rights that he enjoyed in his prepatient status continue, although sometimes in an attenuated form. No one questions the right of the average patient in the average hospital to write a letter and have a nurse mail it, to receive visitors, to make telephone calls. If he wishes to call his lawyer and change his will or call his broker and change his holdings, no one stands in his way. The hospital does have rules—perhaps he cannot make phone calls after ten o'clock at night, or receive visitors except during two periods daily set aside for visiting —but the rules do not seriously interfere with the civil rights of the patient. If the patient is severely ill or recently out of surgery, his doctor may have written some orders that curtail his rights temporarily —he may not be allowed visitors or use of a phone, he may not even be allowed out of bed. But doctor and patient recognize these limitations as temporary and imposed by medical necessity; when the patient's condition has sufficiently improved, his rights are speedily restored.

If the patient is treated in a municipal hospital, he may find more restrictions on his rights. He may find visitors are allowed on only Wednesdays and Sundays. He will not have a bedside telephone, although there probably will be a telephone booth in the corridor. But although he may grumble at the rules of the hospital, he has little cause for complaint, because he is accepting free or substantially subsidized hospital treatment and, as part of this bargain, has agreed to abide by the hospital's rules. His alternative remains—to enter a private hospital, where he will be charged more but be less bound by restrictions.

When a patient enters any psychiatric hospital, he finds that many of his civil rights have been taken away from him. Although the structure of the hospital may be more like the structure of life outside the hospital than he had expected (he may wear ordinary clothes, eat in a cafeteria, work in a hospital office), a whole set of rules may be imposed that resemble those of the correctional institution more than those of the hospital. He may not be allowed to see any visitors, to receive letters from relatives or friends, to reach business associates, or to keep his driver's license.

He may even find that handcuffs can be put on his wrists or a strait-jacket around him, or that he can be held down and forcibly restrained by hospital attendants or locked up in a seclusion room. He may find that he can be sedated and tranquilized by injection in spite of the fact that he is adamant about not wanting to be medicated. If he is less violent, he may be requested to work without pay, or with very little pay, in a hospital kitchen or laundry or on a hospital farm; the request carries teeth since noninterest in work—or even in occupational therapy "busywork"—indicates that the patient is not "really motivated to get well," and the hospital staff will treat him accordingly.

Restrictions on the mental patient will usually be imposed with no distinction between voluntary and committed patients, and whether in a private or state hospital. The hospital feels justified in imposing these restrictions and obligations on the assumption that the patient, by the nature of his disease, cannot be trusted with the civil liberties others enjoy and may have to be required to do things that he does not wish to do but are in his own best interest. In recent years, innovations such as open wards, democratic patient councils, informal admissions, which give the patient the right to leave the hospital without notice, indicate a trend away from coercion, but the trend has not gone far.

Of the state psychiatric hospital, Dr. James Peal says:

The classical state hospital is designed for a custodial contained operation, with descending vertical lines of communication, *i.e.*, control from the top. The attitudes and value systems of the staff have been developed and nurtured by this framework to provide benevolent and enlightened custody. A thorough-going system of rewards and punishments, sanctions, approvals and disapprovals are aspects of the establishment which permit the staff to maintain a *status quo*, with the goal of a smooth-running, trouble-free institution. Medical and other professionals have given sanction to this order of things, in which electroshock therapy, restraint and seclusion, privileges, etc. are aspects of the maintenance of this system. The very effectiveness of this system forms a hard core of resistance to change.[1]

The Report of the American Bar Foundation notes that in 1950 the Council of State Governments expressly stated that the personal rights of mental patients should be protected and the hospitalization should be considered therapeutic rather than punitive. *"Patients while in a hospital should be protected in the enjoyment of personal rights to the extent consistent with required treatment and detention.* This principle is based on the very simple . . . idea that an individual hospitalized for mental illness is only sick. The principle goes beyond such obvious matters as the right to receive visitors and to communicate with relatives, public officials, and others."[2]

Comments the Report:

An examination of the state statutes and administrative regulations indicates, however, that the right to receive visitors or to correspond with persons outside the institution is not generally recognized. Moreover, only a small minority of states have statutes regulating the use of mechanical restraints, of certain kinds of medical treatment, or of patients as hospital employees. The divergence between the statement of the Council of State Governments and existing statutory provisions probably is due to the fact that only in recent times, due to advances in treatment, has "insanity" come generally to be regarded simply as an illness, similar to physical illness. In the past, practically all mentally disabled persons were believed incapable of comprehending or exercising their personal rights. It would be equally foolhardy to say, on the other hand, that in modern times mental patients ought to retain all their personal rights. Effective treatment in many instances necessitates a withdrawal of the patient's rights. The crux of the problem is the extent to which discretion to control the patient's freedom should be placed in the hands of the hospital authorities.[3]

Logically and legally, the rights of a hospitalized patient should depend on whether the patient is a voluntary or a committed patient and whether he is in a general or a licensed psychiatric hospital. But the distinction between the voluntary and the committed patient, as we have seen, usually ceases when the admission procedure is completed; often the only real distinction—for whatever it is worth—is the right of the voluntary patient to leave a certain number of days after having given notice, if the hospital does not move successfully to have him committed in the intervening time.

The distinction between the rights of patients in a general hospital and a licensed psychiatric hospital is more crucial in determining the restraints and restrictions that can legally be imposed. A voluntary psychiatric patient in a general hospital (to which only voluntary patients can be admitted) has the right and ability, if ambulatory, to leave the ward, make telephone calls, write letters, buy stamps, see his lawyer; he has the right to do all these things and others just as if he were a medical patient in the same hospital, subject only to reasonable hospital rules. The hospital has no authority to restrain him or regulate his activities except to the extent that any other patient in the hospital with no psychiatric illness can be restrained and regulated. The hospital cannot require the patient to accept medications against his will, be restrained with handcuffs or camisole, be locked in a seclusion room, be forced or expected to mop the floor, work in the hospital cafeteria, type letters in the hospital superintendent's office, or make beds in the hospital superintendent's home. In every state, there are licensed private psychiatric hospitals and state psychiatric hospitals that are by statute empowered to hold voluntary or committed patients, and while holding them curtail their rights in much the same way that prison inmates' rights are curtailed—to hold the patient against his will, control him, restrain him, and punish and discipline him. In every case, these special licensed psychiatric hospitals or state psychiatric hospitals operate under more scrutiny and supervision by the state authorities than general hospitals, in the hope that this will keep patients from suffering as a result of the diminution of their rights.

In Pennsylvania, for example, Article II, section 201 of the Mental Health Act[4] lists 23 state hospitals where psychiatric patients shall be cared for, and also authorizes other private institutions, which have procured licenses from the Department of Welfare, to care for psychiatric patients; but general hospitals are allowed only to secure licenses for the temporary care of mental patients. In actual practice, general hospitals usually do not secure licenses even for the temporary care of mental patients, because they do not want to be under the special supervision of the Department of Welfare and subject to the requirements for reports to and examinations by that Department, and therefore they restrict admissions to voluntary patients only and operate on the same basis with voluntary psychiatric patients—if they admit such—as with voluntary medical or surgical patients.

Lebensohn[5] has said that there are over 800 psychiatric units in general hospitals in the United States and that these units now admit more patients annually (although they do not compare in number of patient days) than all the public mental hospitals combined. He states that the psychiatric unit of the general hospital has many advantages; in particular, it returns psychiatry to the fold of medicine. Pokorny[6] states that maintaining psychiatric patients in a general hospital usually means that there must be at least a partly locked ward. The question whether many of the patients treated in the psychiatry units of general hospitals are restrained or regulated only to the same extent that the voluntary medical or surgical patient is, or whether extra legal restraints are imposed, does not appear to have received attention.

RIGHT OF COMMUNICATION

The right to use a telephone both to summon help if a patient feels that he is unjustly held, or to keep in touch with friends and family if he does not feel that he is unjustly held, is a right that is of great importance to the mental patient. In earlier days the right to send letters had the same importance; today the right to write letters has a legal importance, since letters can become evidence in a court proceeding, but telephone usage often has more immediate meaning.

These rights to use telephones and write letters, plus the right to have visitors, have sometimes been grouped under the heading of the right to communication. The telephone has not been the subject of any statutory law, but 32 jurisdictions have some statutory law regarding correspondence and 20 have laws regarding visitation.

Some states have viewed the right to send letters as an unlimited right; others have limited it to patients in private institutions; still others have stated that there is such a right but "at the discretion of the hospital superintendent"; and still others have regarded this right to apply only to communications with those persons who would be concerned with the unlawful detention of the patient, such as his lawyer, the commissioner of mental health of the state, or the governor of the State. Connecticut provides that the patient "may correspond with any suitable person"; Georgia and Tennessee that patients are "entitled to communicate by sealed mail or otherwise with persons including official agencies inside or outside the hospital." But Kentucky gives this right only to patients who enter the hospital under a voluntary procedure; Louisiana only at the physician's discretion; and Massachusetts permits the hospital to readdress incoming or outgoing mail to the patient's parent, guardian, or most interested friend.[7]

The Report of the American Bar Foundation points out the relationship between the right of correspondence and the right to a writ of habeas corpus, the most essential of the rights of a hospitalized patient.

Since the power of the hospital to deny the patient visitation or correspondence rights may be misused to the point of depriving him of his right to a writ of habeas corpus, this type of provision is extremely important to the patient. In two New York cases, the state hospital's failure to forward letters to attorneys was held to constitute an unreasonable restraint on the patient's right to a writ of habeas corpus.

In both cases the hospital superintendent—who had the authority to, and in fact did, restrict correspondence—knew that the letters were to an attorney and knew also that they related to habeas corpus proceedings. Although New York patients at that time did not have a right to unrestricted correspondence with an attorney, they did have a right to correspond with the governor, attorney general, judges, district attorneys, and officers of the Department of Mental Hygiene. In the earlier of these two cases, the court, explaining that the exceptions were too restrictive, said:

"Depriving a person confined in a large institution . . . of the right to send a letter to a lawyer . . . imposes an unreasonable restraint upon him never contemplated by the law. . . ."

New York, as a result of these cases, now provides by statute that mental patients have a right to unrestricted correspondence with attorneys from the county in which the patient resides. Colorado, Illinois, Kentucky, Louisiana, Pennsylvania, Texas, and Wisconsin are the only other states that have similar statutory provisions. The failure of the remaining states to enact such provisions opens the way to the same kind of abuse pointed out in the New York cases.[8]

The concept that incoming or outgoing mail should be restricted or censored is based on the idea that incoming letters may be harmful to the patient's mental state and outgoing letters may contain material obscene, libelous, litigious, or disturbing to the recipient. The idea has been expressed that psychotic patients who express delusional ideas in letters would be embarrassed by the contents of these letters after their recovery. Whether patients should be shielded from the outside world and the outside world shielded from patients as part of therapy is questionable; open ward hospitals, which were pioneered in England and have become more accepted in the United States in recent years, do not appear to have any particular problems or any reported lawsuits rising out of the unrestricted flow of mail.

Some hospitals have the policy of not releasing the name of any hospitalized mental patient except to lawyer or relative, on the theory that the mere fact that one is a patient in a psychiatric hospital is stigmatizing, may lead to loss of job or other detriment, and can be withheld as confidential material that falls within the status of privileged communications, in the same way that a lawyer in some instances has the right not to reveal the name of his client. The Report of the American Bar Foundation cites the administrative regulations of Wisconsin's Mendota State Hospital, which, besides forbidding the posting of mail that contains obscene material, threats, statements that might embarrass the patient or his family, and unreliable comments concerning discharge, also prohibit the posting of letters that contain the names of other patients. While such a regulation ostensibly is in the service of the patient population, hospitals do not prohibit their staffs from discussing patients outside the hospital, and if an especially prominent person becomes a patient the fact is often quickly publicized in a community. The policy of no censorship of incoming and outgoing mail, such as that proposed by the British Royal Commission on the Law Relating to Mental Illness, would not appear to do any particular disservice to patients, and it would ensure that one part of the right of communications was not restricted. It would also mean that a time-consuming staff function in state hospitals, censorship of mail, would be unnecessary, and that staff time could be devoted to more therapeutic activities.

The Draft Act prepared as a model under the auspices of the National Institute of Mental Health does not go so far as the recommendation of the British Royal Commission. The Royal Commission recommended "that there should be no censorship of out-going letters from patients . . . except at the request of individual addressees who ask for letters addressed to themselves to be scrutinized or withheld because they find them distressing."[9] The Draft Act recommendation leaves discretion in the hands of hospital administrations, and states that all patients are "entitled to communicate by sealed mail or otherwise . . . subject to the general rules and regulations of the hospital and except to the extent that the head of the hospital determines that it is necessary for the medical welfare of the patient to impose restrictions. . . ."[10]

Even when the patient is given the right to send uncensored mail, if he does not have access to pen, paper and a stamp, his right can be subject to the control of the hospital staff, and as authorities have pointed out, the final decision in an overcrowded and understaffed hospital is often in the hand of a subordinate hospital employee, often nonmedically trained. Only twelve states have statutes designed to see that the patient has access to writing materials and stamps. Georgia requires that all the letters of patients in private asylums only are to be mailed by the patient in a United States post-office box. Rhode Island requires that the patient shall be provided every facility for making communications by mail. Washington requires that materials shall be furnished to the patient for writing at least one letter each week.[11] Pennsylvania gives and withholds the right in the same statutory provision[12]; every patient has the right to be furnished with writing materials and reasonable opportunity, in the discretion of the superintendent, for communicating with any person outside of the institution. "Communications shall be stamped and mailed." The fact that hospital authority has discretion makes this a dubious "right."

Four states have foreseen that a hospital inmate might have the right to send letters to designated persons or to be furnished with writing materials, yet might not, because of ignorance of the fact that they possess such a right, exercise the right. Concerning their laws on written communications, Georgia, Montana, Rhode Island and South Dakota provide that a notice of the statutory right must be posted in the institution, but once again the Georgia law relates to private asylums only.[13]

The right to have visitors is the subject of statutes in 20 jurisdictions, but these statutes do little to make sure that the right is observed, because in most cases it is subject to the discretionary power of the hospital administration. The Draft Act and nine states[14] that have adopted this section of the Draft Act state that patients are "entitled to receive visitors subject to the general rules and regulations of the hospital and except to the extent that the head of the hospital determines that it is necessary for the medical welfare of the patient to impose restrictions." Like many of the statutes on the right to send and receive mail, these statutes on the right to have visitors guarantee rights and withhold them at the same time; the right is dependent on the discretion of the hospital authority and there is no standard set or system of review provided to ensure that the hospital authority is not arbitrary or negligent. Three states—Georgia, Indiana, and Tennessee —have statutes providing that there shall be no discrimination between patients in the same hospital regarding the right to have visitors: "every patient is entitled to receive visitors during regular visiting hours." Five states are concerned with the right to be visited by ministers: Iowa specifies that "patients are to be allowed at least one hour each Sunday to receive spiritual advice from any recognized clergyman who represents their religious belief," and Kentucky provides a fine if the patient's right to see a minister is denied.[15] Seven states provide that the patient has the right to see his legal counsel[16]; his right to see others is discretionary. Connecticut's statute reads, for example: "visits by any member of the family, relative or friend are allowed if the superintendent does not think they will be injurious, if approved by the welfare commissioner, or if ordered by the court."[17]

A few states have special provisions allowing the patient to be treated by his own physician for nonpsychiatric conditions while he is in the hospital. A right of patient specified in the Pennsylvania statute is "To be visited and examined at all reasonable hours by any medical or osteopathic practitioner designated by him or any member of his family or 'near friend'; with the consent of the patient and of the Superintendent, the medical or osteopathic practitioner may attend the patient for all maladies other than mental illness in the same manner as if the patient were in his own home."[18] Since this right is discretionary on the part of the Superintendent and no patients are informed that they possess this right, this law has little if any application. Ohio's statute is more forthright: "The patient's personal physician shall be admitted at all times."[19]

Some of the hospitals most restrictive concerning visitors—who deny them absolutely to certain patients as part of their treatment program and only allow other patients to have visitors during certain very restricted visiting times—paradoxically, also try to encourage volunteers to come to see hospital patients on the grounds that maintaining contact with the "outside world" is important for patients and in line with the theory that impaired interpersonal relationships may be a factor in the progress of mental disease. Many patients, who would be willing to visit with their own friends or relatives, but who do not wish to visit with a student nurse or a volunteer, are labelled as uncooperative and difficult, in the same way that patients who resent the tasks assigned to them in occupational therapy—although their resentment may be a sign of good reality testing and good ego strength—are labelled as having a poor prognosis.

RIGHT TO PURSUE LEGAL REMEDIES

The right of communication, either by mail, telephone, or having visitors, has been stressed not only because it is important to the patient socially but because it relates to his ability to secure his own release from the hospital if he is improperly held. A patient who has been improperly hospitalized or who has been properly hospitalized but now feels he is well enough to be discharged has open one main avenue of recourse—an appeal to the courts. This appeal may be in the form of a request for a judicial discharge, provided for in 33 states, or an application for a writ of habeas corpus, allowed in all states. In either case, the request or the application goes to the courts, where the questions of improper commitment or improper retention of the patient can be heard. For most patients, the legal procedures involved are complex, and even the fact that these legal avenues are open may be unknown; they therefore depend on advice of counsel. Counsel does not always respond to a plea from a hospital patient; often lawyers do not wish to become involved: they may feel that if the patient is in a mental hospital, the problem may be too complicated or too unremunerative to warrant their involvement. But whether or not he responds, counsel should at least receive the plea of the hospital patient.

In its law concerning rights of patients, Pennsylvania spells out this aspect of the law unequivocally and clearly.[20] All patients have the right "to communicate with and to be alone at any interview with his counsel or representative of the department [of welfare], and to send sealed communications to the superintendent, the department, the court, if any, which committed him, and the Governor." Thus every person with the power to free the patient from the hospital may be sent sealed mail, and the lawyer who can advise in the attempt for freedom can visit. But only six other states[21]—Connecticut, Louisiana, Massachusetts, Ohio, Rhode Island and Vermont—have provisions about the right to visitation by counsel (there is no method of making sure that the patient knows that he does have this basic right) and only six additional states give the patient the statutory right to write to counsel.[22] Even in these states, there is no requirement in the law that a patient be informed of these rights to communicate with and be visited by counsel.

OTHER RIGHTS

Besides the rights of communication and to pursue legal remedies to forestall improper hospitalization, other rights are applicable to mental patients that are not involved in ordinary hospitalizations. One is the right to be free or reasonably free of mechanical restraints; another is a theoretical "right" to be treated; a third is the right to be compensated for work done while in the hospital.

MECHANICAL RESTRAINTS

Mechanical restraints were widely used at one time. In England in 1815, a parliamentary investigation focused attention on the extent and the character of the restraints used on patients. Fifty years later, Dr. John Connelly, superintendent of the Middlesex Asylum, published his *The Treatment of the Insane without Mechanical Restraints*. He advocated kindness, patience and understanding on the part of the staff, the removal of prison-like and punitive aspects of hospitalization, and emphasis on recreational and occupational activities. Although Connelly's book led to reforms in England, it had little influence in this country. American psychiatrists, considering the question of the abolition of mechanical restraints, emphasized the increased number of personnel that would be necessary to handle patients and even American patriotism was cited as a reason for continuing restraints. As Deutsch has said, it was argued that "the patients in European institutions, accustomed as they were to unquestioned acceptance of authority, might willingly submit to 'moral' restraint, but not your liberty-loving American who, sane or insane, would never agree placidly to the imposition of authority by an individual."[23]

Restraints were abolished or almost abolished in a few American hospitals, and sometimes these were the very hospitals where cure rates (based on discharge percentages) were highest. Lebensohn has written:

> One can find records of hospitals which abolished restraint, unlocked doors, and developed within the hospital an effective and to some extent democratic society . . . and then the Superintendent retired or died; in ten years' time the doors were locked again, the padded rooms were in use, new strait jackets bought, and the hospital was back where it was before that Superintendent had created this therapeutic community.[24]

Since the era of tranquilizers, restraints have much less usefulness than they once had. But practically all workers in the field feel that there are times when a patient is so self-destructive, assaultive, or over-active that restraints may be necessary. Restraints have been used sometimes as a punishment, and in large hospitals they are imposed at the will of ward attendants without effective supervision of medical staff. Says the Report of the American Bar Foundation[25]:

Unless the use of physical restraint becomes so infrequent that the physician can check each case, it is difficult to see how a patient can be protected against possible abuses.

The requirement that a restraint order be ordered on the patient's clinical record is designed to protect such abuses. The success of this procedure is dependent, however, on who may see the record and on his authority. A look at protective measures in other countries would be enlightening at this point. In England and Wales, full particulars concerning restraints must be reported in a medical certificate; and reports of restraint are sent quarterly from the hospital to the Board of Control, a central agency supervising the practices of all institutions. Norway also requires that quarterly reports on restraint be sent to a control commission. The periodic report to an outside agency would seem to afford better protection to the patient against unauthorized use of physical restraints than a mere entry in his clinical record, which may go unnoticed.

Even when restraint is absolutely necessary, there still remain questions of patients' rights with respect to the means and duration of restraint. Among the physical restraints used in mental institutions are muffs, straps, belts and wristlets, camisoles, dry packs, lock chairs, and sheet restraints. Restraint by fear of 'soap-socking', 'toweling', and 'ducking' are also practiced. Some of these are more confining and dehumanizing than others. A strap on one arm, for example, might provide sufficient restraint and at the same time would leave the patient free to perform functions, while another type of restraint might totally immobilize him. Obviously, there is no justification for the use of a greater amount of restraint than is necessary to prevent the patient from committing destructive physical acts.

Eleven states have statutes providing for use of mechanical restraints. In eight of these—Georgia, Idaho, Missouri, New Mexico, North Dakota, Oklahoma, Pennsylvania, and Utah—it is not clear whether the law was designed to ensure that only medical authorities would order restraints—"determination of need is to be made by the head of the hospital or his designee"—or to relieve doctors of liability if there should be an action against them after restraints are used. Kansas specifies that "restraints are to be applied only if prescribed by a physician." Massachusetts law is clearer:

Restraint is to be applied only in the presence of the superintendent, the physician, or an assistant physician on his written order. In the case of an emergency it may be applied in the physician's absence or without a written order but immediately after the imposition of the restraint, its use is to be reported to the physician who is to investigate the case and approve or disapprove the restraint imposed. Restraints are to be imposed only in cases of extreme violence, infliction of self-injury, active homicidal or suicidal condition or physical exhaustion.

Texas law specifies that "restraints are to be applied only if prescribed by a physician and are to be removed as soon as possible."

The North Dakota statute, uniquely, in addition to the statutory authorization of restraints cited above, also says, "Any person having the care of a mentally ill person and restraining such person, either with or without authority, who shall treat such person with wanton severity, harshness, or cruelty, or who shall abuse such person in any way, shall be guilty of a misdemeanor and will be liable in an action for damages."[26]

The eleven states that have statutes governing the use of mechanical restraints and one state without such a statute—Kentucky—require that the hospital record show the reason for the use of the restraint. There is no such requirement in other jurisdictions.

RIGHT TO TREATMENT

Until very recent years almost no attention was paid by psychiatrists or lawyers to profound questions about the hospitalized patient's right to treatment, his right to compensation for work done for the hospital, his right to be free of the necessity of working for the hospital. Patients who are not dangerous to themselves or others committed to state hospitals for treatment often receive little or no treatment except, if it is a form of treatment, custodial care. Birnbaum has made the revolutionary proposal that these patients have a moral right—and potentially a legal right—either to be treated or discharged.

I have advocated the recognition and enforcement of the legal right of a mentally disordered inmate of a public mental institution to adequate medical treatment for his mental disorder. For convenience, I have called this concept the right to treatment. At the present time, although our society undoubtedly recognizes a moral right to treatment, our courts have never decided whether there is a legal right to treatment.
The concepts underlying the advocacy of the right to treatment are that being mentally disordered is not a crime; that if the state involuntarily institutionalizes a mentally disordered person because he is sufficiently mentally disordered to require institutionalization, then the state owes a duty to provide this person with reasonable medical care; that if it fails to do so then the person is virtually a prisoner, rather than a patient; and, that to treat him as a prisoner is depriving him of his liberty without due process of law.[27]

The arbitrary quality of the decision to hospitalize or not to hospitalize an individual patient is emphasized in some of his statistics; citing psychiatric hospital residency rates per 100,000 population varying from 92 in Utah to 767 in the District of Columbia, he has stated:

> . . . it is often social and not legal or medical factors that are the primary causes of these variations. . . . As the admission, resident-inmate, and discharge rates in our state mental institutions vary from place to place and from time to time, it indicates that there are many severely mentally ill persons who, in a certain community and at a certain time, would not be committed and would be allowed to remain in the community. These same persons, however, in another community or at another time, would be committed after a finding they require—voluntarily or involuntarily—institutional care and treatment. . . .[28]

The views of Birnbaum and of others who feel that the mentally ill have a right to be treated possibly represent less an attempt to get recognition for a new legal principle than a desire to focus the attention of the public and the legislatures on the lack of personnel and the inadequacy of the therapeutic approach in most state hospitals.

The Report of the American Bar Foundation documents the lack of therapeutic care and even of diagnostic labeling in some state hospitals. A study of Texas mental institutions showed that 70% of the patients—particularly the elderly—did not require hospital care, and, on the other hand, patients in the hospital who needed care were neglected. Of 134 patients in one ward, 45 had never been diagnosed and this condition prevailed throughout the state with 30% of all patients lacking a diagnosis. The Report quotes the American Psychiatric Association to the effect that discharges from mental hospitals are directly proportional to the size of their staffs. It concludes:

> . . . that understaffed institutions not only fail to detect and prevent improper hospitalizations but prove of little positive value to the patient once he has been admitted. Patients who, if given the proper treatment, would ordinarily recover tend to become instead permanent state wards whose mental condition, if anything, is less satisfactory than it was when they originally entered the institution. Moreover, poorly staffed hospitals are often unable to take the necessary steps to discover those who have improved under institutional care and perhaps are ready for discharge.[29]

But the fact that mental hospitals are understaffed has not been considered up to this time primarily a legal problem, and if patients have a right to good therapy and a right to be hospitalized where there is a sufficient staff for correct diagnosis and prompt discharge when cured, then understaffing may be a problem more for the legislature than for the courts.

WORK FOR PATIENTS

The employment of mental patients in state hospitals—where they act as cooks, bakers, gardeners, wash the cars of staff members, sometimes work as help in homes of members of the staff on the hospital grounds, and perform numerous other functions—has long been an integral part of the state hospital system.

Pinel, in his *Treatise on Insanity*, which was published shortly after his dramatic freeing of the enchained patients at the time of the French Revolution, advocated work for mental patients, although he did not necessarily advocate that they perform the dull and unrewarding work of the hospital.

> In all public asylums as well as in prisons and hospitals, the surest, and, perhaps, the only method of securing health, good order, and good manners, is to carry into decided and habitual execution the natural law of bodily labour, so contributive and essential to human happiness. This truth is especially applicable to lunatic asylums: and I am convinced that no useful and durable establishment of that kind can be founded excepting on the basis of interesting and laborious employment. I am very sure that few lunatics, even in their most furious state, ought to be without some active occupation. . . . Laborious employment . . . is not a little calculated to divert the thoughts of lunatics from their usual morbid channel, to fix their attention upon more pleasing objects, and by exercise to strengthen the functions of the understanding.[30]

The USSR has led the world in advocating the use of sheltered workshops, combined with drug therapy, to return mental patients to the normal world; a national policy for rehabilitating the mentally ill calls for workshops which are outpatient rehabilitation centers to be connected with mental hospitals. Organizational models have been developed for individualized workshops in communities of different sizes and socioeconomic character. A master plan has been adapted for both agricultural and industrial areas. Industries are required by law to find jobs for rehabilitated mental patients. The Russian program is based on statements of two of its most eminent scientists. Pavlov once wrote, "The best remedy for disturbances of higher nervous activity is mechanical and physical work. Help is possible if physical work corresponding to the individual's potentialities is correctly applied." And Korsakoff wrote, "One of the most powerful motivations is that of activity, of knowledge. In hospitals for the mentally ill, many are deprived of the possibility of satisfying this urge. Owing to idleness, their mental energy wanes and the purposeless passing of time leads to degradation. Systematic, meaningful occupations have a beneficial influence not only on those chronically ill with persistent and progressive mental debility but also on acute patients, giving an outlet for energies that otherwise would be manifested in destruction and anxiety."[31]

Two psychiatrists at Ohio State University have questioned the value of occupational therapy on the basis of a study of acutely ill mental patients in an intensive-treatment hospital. Female patients were assigned at random into groups receiving daily occupational therapy of one hour, therapy of three hours, work in dining room or offices of a half-hour—or none of these. None of the groups showed any major differences in improved functioning.[32] One of the authors noted that this was the first time a study of this kind had been done "despite the fact that we spend millions of dollars for occupational therapy every year." A major difference between the therapy involved in this experiment and the USSR program is that the latter is designed to provide meaningful work and to serve as a transition between the hospital and the working world.

Private hospitals are staffed by maids, dining room or cafeteria workers, secretarial help and other forms of outside labor; in state hospitals much of this work is done by the patients themselves. The claim is often made that the jobs now being performed by state hospital patients are therapeutic for the patients, but the question has been raised why staff of private hospitals do not utilize this kind of therapy to the same degree. The chief reason for the employment of mental patients in the hospital seems to be economic, to bring down the cost per day to the state of maintaining psychiatric patients: these patients by tradition have not been expected to pay the cost of their own hospitalization, and hospitalization insurance plans have usually expressly excluded the costs of mental hospitalization.

The employment of hospital patients to perform hospital functions is usually not voluntary: it is compulsory, and the question has been asked recently in two different forms whether patients' rights are infringed when they are forced to work. One question concerns the rate of pay that patients receive and whether they have been or are being exploited, the other whether hospital administrators tend to allow good workers to remain in the hospital after the point in their recovery where ordinarily they would be discharged. Statutes on the subject throw little light on the problem. "In general it is unclear whether the purpose of statutes authorizing patient labor is to provide occupational and vocational therapy for the patients . . . or whether it is to provide free labor for the institution. . . . In addition, most statutes fail to provide a clear answer to the question of payment for the patient's work."[33]

The Council of State Governments in its survey of mental health programs found that only one-third of the hospitals surveyed paid the patients for their labor, and probably none of these paid more than token—sometimes called "symbolic"—wages. Goldman and Ross[34] have charged that many patients work ten to 14 hours a day for little or no pay. It is safe to say that patients working in state hospitals receive neither the minimum wage stipulated by federal law nor the pay that an outsider would receive for doing comparable work. As a result, the cost of hospitalizing patients in a mental hospital in some states is as little as $4.54 a day, compared to costs of $30 or $35 a day in private mental hospitals and more than $41 daily for medical and surgical patients.[35]

The Council of State Governments concluded that there was no real problem in this sphere:

Obviously, no hospital worthy of the name would use this situation exploitatively in relation to the patient. No hospital worthy of the name would regard a patient as a source of cheap or free labor, nor would it assign a patient to work except in his own interest and in an occupation that was suitable for him in view of his condition and his requirements.[36]

This denial of the problem hardly helps. Whether or not hospitals that do exploit hospital labor are worthy of their name, there is no doubt that the use of patient labor is the main factor in the low cost per day of mental hospitalization, and that this is in the interest of the patient is doubtful.

F. Lewis Bartlett, a psychiatrist who has had hospital experience in Kentucky and Pennsylvania, has led a campaign against the use of patient labor on the ground not that the patient is financially exploited but that state hospitals have as their main orientation the concept of economic self-sufficiency and minimum cost to the state and that therefore the concept of optimum patient care has only lip service paid to it. Dr. Bartlett has described[37] a four-man team of patients that he trained and utilized when he was a psychiatry resident in a state hospital. These patients assisted in giving electric shock therapy and were on call to handle patient emergencies. They were given armbands designating them as "First Aider," and were domiciled in double rooms instead of on a ward. They were also given a fifty-cent canteen card weekly in exchange for their seven-day-a-week duties.

Only after I was away from the state mental hospital for a while, however, and could view my use of the First Aiders in some perspective did I come to realize that this really represented a gross abdication of my primary responsibility as a psychiatrist. The recompenses I arranged for the First Aiders may very well have led them to consider me a good guy. But as an integral part of the hospital, whose interests came first, I was actually being a very poor doctor to them; they were helping me with masses of other patients while their need for recovery and discharge was completely overlooked. Their role of institutional worker was so established and self-effacing and accepted that the question of their further recovery never came up.

Dr. Bartlett says that State hospitals use up to 75% of patients as workers on the hospital farm, in the dairy, on the grounds, in carpenter shops, kitchens, dining rooms, and laundries, in the wards, in maintenance and engineering.

Unfortunately, this exploitation can be accommodating to their illness and increase their dependency on the institution. Rather than getting well, they can become 'good patients,' and their hospital stays stretch into years. Tragically, without such institutional peonage on the part of its patients, the state mental hospital system would have to close down completely.

He recommends that patients by statute be given the right to fair payment for nontherapeutic labors.

The expense of paying the patients, or employees, rather than depending on institutional peonage, would increase the immediate out-of-pocket costs of running these so-called hospitals. But the institutions would then have no need for any patient or his work, and restructuring will have already started. The next step would be the hiring of adequate doctors and staff to inhibit pathological dependency on the institution, to effect recoveries and separations, and reduce substantially hospital populations.

Like the right to adequate therapy, the right to just compensation for work performed is not recognized in any jurisdiction, but there may be increasing demands in the future, on the theory that mental illness is a disease, for legislation to ensure that mental patients are treated like other patients instead of like prisoners, whose prison farm-and-work situation so closely resembles the state hospital patient-labor system.

PERIODIC EXAMINATIONS

Concerning the termination of hospitalization, the Report of the American Bar Foundation states: "No one will argue with the proposition that a patient should have an absolute right to discharge when his condition no longer warrants hospitalization."[38] But this right is based on another right, the right of periodic examinations. If a hospital is so understaffed that patients are not well known to hospital staff members and are not examined thoroughly at frequent intervals, the conditions requiring hospitalization may be terminated but the patient will linger in the hospital. Only nine states specify that patients must receive a postadmission examination and only 12 require periodic examinations thereafter. The frequency set forth in the statute is not less often than every three months in Tennessee, six months in four other states, yearly in two, and "as frequently as necessary" or "as practicable" (in the words of the Arizona statute) in four others; New York's revised mental hygiene code provides for examinations at varying intervals, initially six months, next one year, and thereafter every two years. Says the Report: "an adequate enforcement of this right should receive the attention of legislators, not only in terms of prescribed duties for hospital authorities but also of the establishment of facilities and medical staffs sufficient to discharge these duties."[39]

The psychiatric hospital patient undoubtedly has the right to good custodial care even if his right to good therapy is at present doubtful. Hospitals have the responsibility of seeing that suicidal patients are protected from their own impulses, and that patients are protected from other hazards that can be anticipated, including assault by other patients. A New York case involved the suicide of an escaped mental patient. The state was held liable for damages for the suicide because the escape was held to have been made possible by negligent hospital supervision and the hospital knew that the patient had suicidal tendencies.[40] And the New York Court of Claims has ruled that a child born as the result of the rape of a patient in Manhattan State Hospital by another patient can recover damages for being brought into life, in addition to the damages his mother can claim if negligence on the part of the hospital can be established.[41]

In 1962, the annual conference of State Mental Health Authorities with the Surgeon General issued a plea for the purging of "any statement of discrimination pertaining to the mentally ill from present laws."[42] The conference recommended that rights of mental patients should include the confidentiality of clinical and court records to avoid job and other discriminations and prevent such discriminations as the termination of auto insurance by virtue of mental hospitalization. "No patient should lose any civil rights solely by virtue of hospitalization for a mental illness," recommended the conference. It listed as methods by which rights are frequently abrogated: automatic suspension of driver's license; automatic loss of legal competency; loss of old-age benefits under the Social Security Act and Federal public assistance. It also recommended that private health-insurance prepayment plans be prohibited from discriminating against mental patients by excluding them from hospitalization benefits.

At present the hospitalized mental patient has few rights guaranteed by statute. He usually does not have the right to demand a psychiatric examination on admission or a periodic examination after admission. He does not have the right in many jurisdictions to have his records kept confidential if he is a state hospital patient. He does not have the right in most jurisdictions to send uncensored mail to those in authority who might obtain his release if he is being held illegally. In these and many other respects, he is dealt with more like a prisoner than a patient. The right of a writ of habeas corpus, so that his case can be considered on its merits in a public court, remains his ultimate right; but without the right of easy access to legal counsel, that right has only partial effectiveness. Moreover, many patients have no understanding of the nature of this right and how to obtain it for themselves.

Most patients who are in mental hospitals probably belong there. In many urban areas, because psychiatric hospitals are so overcrowded, patients who seek admission because they are hallucinating are often treated with tranquilizers and sent home. The problem of patients who should be hospitalized and are not is probably immeasurably more serious than that of patients who should not be hospitalized but are. Nevertheless, the right of hospitalized patients to be discharged when appropriate should not be a quasiright, dependent on the discretion and good will of hospital staffs and on the need of hospitals to discharge old patients to make way for new patients. It should be a real right, based on legislative safeguards and diligence on the part of lawyers in seeing that these safeguards are observed.

CHAPTER 15

Quasi Criminals: Juvenile Offender, Sexual Psychopath

A DOMINANT legal theme, as we know, is that courts will give special protection to the helpless or the unfortunate. They will do more for orphans, illiterates, the mentally deranged or other categories of handicapped persons than they will for the average everyday citizen. When courts depart from their usual methods and procedures to give special help to unfortunates, the result is not always entirely gain. The loss involves the protection of individual rights that have been safeguarded by the centuries-old methods which the courts now abandon. An example is the right to a jury trial; when this right is denied certain categories of patients in "their own best interests," the defendant may or may not receive a benefit.

When the court is concerned with someone who is mentally disabled, it will readily abandon traditional procedures in the hope that the ill person will receive prompt treatment. The court feels easy in modifying its methods—even if some of the protection of the law is lost—because the theoretical goal of the legal procedure is therapy and not punishment. The other extreme is the typical criminal case, where the court is meticulous in seeing that legal safeguards—such as trial by jury, the right to be defended by counsel, bail, knowledge of the charges brought—are accorded the defendant.

The law, however, has not made up its mind about two groups of offenders who are not clearly mentally ill and not typically criminal. By virtue of the type of crime committed and by virtue of immaturity, respectively, the sexual psychopath and the juvenile offender have been treated by the courts as special categories, in reliance on laws that permit them to depart from the traditional criminal procedure and that provide for treatment instead of, or in addition to, punishment.

The desire of the court to place sexual psychopaths in a special category is not entirely altruistic. Many of the laws concerning sexual psychopathy were passed in the heat of public reaction to the commission of a flagrant sexual crime or the sometimes greater heat aroused by a series of "minor" sexual misdemeanors. Courts are not sure what to do with sexual offenders and they are not happy in dealing with them. Theoretically, a rational bank robber who serves ten years in prison will see the error of his ways, and rob no more; equally theoretically, the irrational sexual criminal will probably leave jail undeterred by his experience, and repeat his crime. Although authorities debate whether sexual criminals are more likely to continue to repeat their offenses—or, to use the language of the penologists, to be recidivists—the courts feel more secure if they can turn these offenders over to the psychiatrist for treatment and to be held until they are "cured."

Juveniles too, for somewhat different reasons, are felt to need treatment and to require being held not for a stated period of time but until they are either "cured" or have graduated from the ranks of juveniles.

These two groups, accordingly, have been given a special status before the law, which has been hailed as a humane advance because it recognizes the psychological determinants in criminal activities, and because it proposes therapy rather than punishment as the means of preventing such criminal activities in the future. Recently, questions have been asked increasingly of the effectiveness as well as the humanity of this special approach.

THE SEXUAL CRIMINAL

One problem has always been whether the sexual criminal constitutes a really separate grouping distinguished from other criminals. Many psychiatrists, particularly those psychoanalytically oriented, believe that psychiatric determinants exist in most or all criminal actions. Sexual excitement appears to be a factor in many crimes: the erotic feelings that accompany such activities as fire-setting have been described in the psychiatric literature, and psychiatrists are familiar with the descriptions of increasing tension and restlessness that culminate in many ostensibly nonsexual crimes varying from passing checks to robbing gasoline stations. When the criminal who suffers from increasing tension expresses it in transvestism, molesting a child, or even rape, it is easy to pin a psychiatric label on him; when the crime is forgery, fraud, or robbery, the sexual motives that may seem apparent to the psychiatrist often elude the court and the jury. Crimes that do not obviously have a sexual motivation are assumed to be the result of deliberate intent; if the accused is wealthy or has a background of intensive psychiatric care, psychiatric testimony may try to show that the act was not criminal as much as psychopathologic, but usually the psychiatrist is involved in court proceedings only when sexual or irrational motivation is obvious.

With their particular point of view, many psychiatrists would wish to have a part in all determinations of guilt or innocence, and many would wish to have a major part in the care of patients who have been convicted of crime, with the aim of rehabilitation by psychiatric therapy. In an earlier period, when optimism concerning the effectiveness of psychotherapy and the treatability of all patients ran higher, some judges did turn much of their responsibility in some criminal cases over to the psychiatrist who was willing to assume the burden. The results were usually not happy. Some judges, disappointed in the results of those psychiatrists, psychologists and social workers who have advised on the disposition of criminal charges and attempted to treat offenders, have reacted against the psychiatric approach entirely. Nevertheless, psychiatric beliefs have had an increasing overall influence in the administration of criminal justice, and some lawyers and some psychiatrists urge an even larger role for the psychiatrist in the judicial process.

Judge Bazelon, for instance, famous as the author of the *Durham* decision, which deals with standards of criminal responsibility, believes that psychiatric treatment in community mental health centers can be the answer to the problem of crime in modern society.[1]

The real hope for stemming crime lies in finding the basic causes of disturbed behavior, David L. Bazelon, Chief Judge of the U. S. Court of Appeals, District of Columbia Circuit, told a conference for leaders in state mental health planning.

"Unless we learn to understand the offender, find out why he committed his crime and remove the causes, the factors which produced him will produce more offenders like him and will produce them faster than we can stuff them into human warehouses," Judge Bazelon said.

Community mental health centers could be the answer, Judge Bazelon said, for the information they provide will not only help the individual, but "help the community to understand the individual."

This approach offers greater hope for reducing crime than increasing the police forces.

However, Judge Bazelon pointed out to the meeting in Washington, D. C., sponsored by the American Psychiatric Association, that although crime is one manifestation of failure and perhaps not the worst, criminal law often avoids inquiring into why an individual's expectations have been disappointed.

Even though criminal offenders and the mentally ill have traditionally received the same "isolation" treatment from the community in large understaffed institutions, "there is more recognition of the need to change methods of treatment for the mentally disabled than for those convicted of crime," he said.

Besides offering an alternative to hospital commitment, Judge Bazelon believes that these centers could offer an alternative to prison commitment.

Although a hard core of offenders and mentally disturbed people require isolated care, most offenders end up in prison "simply because there is no alternative."

The variety of service offered by community mental health centers—day care, night care and after care—could help offenders resolve their problems so that eventually they could "make it" on the outside.

And Dr. Bruno Cormier, assistant professor of psychiatry at McGill University, has recently defined crime as a social illness and asked for a greater role for psychiatry in administering justice. In determining the sentence, the judge must understand the individual criminal, and closer cooperation with the clinician can help him gain this understanding. "Unless judges enlist scientists in human behavior to help . . . it is impossible for justice to be individualized." The psychiatrist would have a part in the judicial process not only in assessing the criminal but also in interpreting the unconscious motives of the judge to the judge. Warning of the danger of retaliation on the part of jurists, Dr. Cormier said, "It is here for psychiatrists to remind the sentencing judge that as long as man is man, retaliation may be present as an unconscious inspiration for punishment."[2]

Not all opinion, legal and psychiatric, would have the psychiatrist take over the role of arbiter of justice as well as healer of criminal tendencies. Dr. Henry Davidson has warned psychiatrists from becoming "Dr. Fixits" even if asked to assume that role by courts in the trial of an emotionally disturbed defendant.[3]

"We must avoid the curious situation existing in some places where the judge feels the defendant is a sick individual to be treated, not a criminal to be punished, and therefore the psychiatrist should take over," he told a symposium at the first Interamerican Conference on Legal Medicine and Forensic Science, which was held in San Juan, Puerto Rico, in 1963. He said that when this occurs psychiatrists may think the judge enlightened. This is sometimes true, but not infrequently "it may simply be that the judge wants to get off a hot spot. He may not know what to do with a sex offender. He does not want to imprison the man, either because of fear that in the one-sex environment of the prison the deviation will worsen or because such a sentence might stamp the judge as old-fashioned. He is afraid to put the defendant on probation lest the offensive behavior continue.

"At this point Dr. Fixit enters the picture. Dr. Fixit is a psychiatrist who has all the answers . . . so the court turns the defendant over to the psychiatrist and with one brilliant stroke the judicial dilemma is solved."

Dr. Davidson said psychiatrists should never forget that "in the minds of the public there does exist a demand that he who deliberately does that which he knows he should not do should suffer for it. If we fashion a responsibility formula that ignores this, we do so at the risk of terminating our usefulness in this field and thus of injuring the sick individuals we are sworn to protect."

Dr. Davidson's conclusion was that "crime is socially defined; it is largely socially determined; it ought to be dealt with by social instruments."

The most intensive involvement by psychiatrists in the realm of criminal justice occurs when they are willing to tell the court that they feel that a convicted offender can be cured by psychiatric treatment, and when the court, as a result, puts the criminal on probation with the psychiatrist in a position of authority over him. The *Philadelphia Inquirer* of January 13, 1962, under the headline "Judge Gold Puts Sex Offender on Probation Again," reports a typical case. The offender, a 24-year-old married male schoolteacher, and a male companion had been accused of sexually molesting two 12-year-old girls. The newspaper story follows:

Confessed sex offender HW, just released from Norristown State Hospital after 90 days of mental examinations, was again placed on 10 years' psychiatric probation Friday by Judge Joseph E. Gold.

In taking that action, the judge quoted the opinions of several psychiatrists that probation was the best way to rehabilitate the 24-year-old former Philadelphia schoolteacher.

The doctors also reported they believed W would not pose a threat to society. His main troubles appeared to be a feeling of inferiority, which led him to commit the act for which he was arrested, the report stated.

W's companion in the assault on two 12-year-old girls last June 21, EG, 23, was returned to Norristown for an indefinite period of not more than one year for psychiatric treatment. This also was done on recommendation of the physicians there.

Except for his 90-day stay at the hospital, W was given the original probation sentence imposed upon him by Judge Gold last September 29 which brought storms of protest to City Hall by many citizens.

Judge Gold, on petition of District Attorney James C. Crumlish, Jr., reconsidered the sentence on Oct. 13, vacated the original probation and sent W to the hospital for further tests. Technically, the judge Friday sentenced W to five months and 10 days in prison—the total time he spent in county prison awaiting trial in the hospital. The sentence, therefore, was already completed and he went free at the end of the court session.

Judge Gold again imposed the 10 years of probation with one minor change —instead of reporting once a month for psychiatric treatment he must report every two weeks. . . .

First Assistant District Attorney Paul M. Chalfin said that the ruling "spoke for itself" and that his office would take no further action in the case.

The report from Norristown was made by Dr. William P. Camp, superintendent of the institution. It agreed with earlier findings by Drs. John G. Torney and Martin F. Hayes, of the Neuropsychiatric Division of Quarter Sessions Court, that W should be put on probation.

Dr. Camp said that W was "not likely to be a threat to society" and that the type of mental treatment needed by him probably could not be obtained in a hospital or a prison.

Judge Gold had been considering sentencing G to one day to life under the Barr-Walker Act for habitual sex criminals. Dr. Camp's report, however, altered his view.

He said that physicians at the hospital felt that the offense and the surrounding conditions "probably do not fit the intent of the Barr-Walker Act in that in practice this has largely been reserved for individuals who are mentally ill or whose acts have been violent and constitute a threat of actual bodily harm to the public."

Instead, Dr. Camp suggested that G's commitment to the hospital should be extended for an indefinite period by the court "so that he may be tried in group psychotherapy for six months to one year."

If this appears to be successful for G, Dr. Camp said it would be reported to the judge.

If G is found unable to improve, the doctor's report continued, then he will be returned to court for other disposition of his case.

W and G had pleaded guilty and were committed to county prison. During that time they were examined by court psychiatrists. Then, on September 29, the two were sentenced—W to probation and G to the hospital for further tests.

It was during the sentencing that Judge Gold stirred up the controversy with a remark to [Assistant District Attorney] Harris, who was about to object to the leniency shown W.

Harris said the girls had suffered a traumatic experience.

"The girls will get over it," observed Judge Gold.

The girls, whose names have been withheld by the *Inquirer*, are West Philadelphia parochial school students. They were walking home from a movie at 11:30 p.m. June 21.

A car containing W and G drove up to them at 53rd St. and Woodland Ave. The men identified themselves as policemen and ordered the girls into the car for being out after the juvenile curfew.

After the girls got into the auto, the pair sped away to a darkened driveway and proceeded to molest both children. Later, the girls were allowed to leave the auto and one of them noted the license number.

It turned out to be W's car—a white Thunderbird. Both men were taken into custody the next day. They were identified by both victims in a hearing in morals court.

As reported, this case raises a number of questions.

1. *Judge Gold's reason for imposing psychiatric probation instead of a jail sentence for W: the opinions of psychiatrists that probation was the best way to rehabilitate him.*

But criminal justice by legislative direction is not designed to be merely rehabilitative; it is also designed to protect society, to be punitive, to provide comparable justice for all accused and a deterring example to potential criminals. The argument that probation rather than jail would be helpful to the criminal would, if applied across the board, keep almost all first offenders and many repeat offenders out of jail and turn this vast number of people over to the psychiatrist as potential patients.

2. *The doctors' report that W would not pose a threat to society, and that his main trouble was a feeling of inferiority.* (The actual text of

the psychiatrists' report: "this man is capable of receiving and profiting from psychotherapy and we would add that he needs this therapy to combat the feelings of inferiority which were a contributory cause of the act of which he was convicted. In our opinion the kind of treatment he needs is intensive, psychoanalytically oriented, long-term psychotherapy which he is not likely to get in a State hospital or a prison. . . .")

This explanation seems scarcely sufficient for the dynamics of impersonating an officer, holding girls against their will, and sexually assaulting them. These actions seem to be indicative of more pathology than the immaturity and sense of inferiority mentioned in the psychiatric report.

3. The striking disparity between the sentences of W, psychiatric probation, and G, who was sent to a state psychiatric hospital for a period of not more than one year but who would then be subject to further sentencing by the court.

No facts were presented during the trial to explain such disparity. The only relevant factors seem to have been the recommendations of the psychiatrists and that a private psychiatrist was willing to undertake the therapy of W.

4. The original probation provision that W must report to his psychiatrist once a month, later changed by Judge Gold, to every two weeks.

Neither time interval is consistent with the "intensive, psychoanalytically oriented, long-term psychotherapy" recommended by the psychiatrists.

5. The inconsistency between Dr. Camp's statement that intensive psychotherapy could not be obtained for W in a state hospital and the fact that the court-imposed frequency of one hour every two weeks does not represent intensive treatment.

Psychoanalytically oriented psychotherapy that is considered intensive is sometimes on the basis of five hours weekly and never on the basis of less than one hour weekly. Of course, Judge Gold's specification represents a minimum, and the private psychiatrist in charge of the case can impose a schedule of more frequent appointments. Then the great problems arise of a psychotherapist with unusual power over the patient. In this case, if the patient refuses to come more frequently, or if he feels the psychiatrist's fee is too high, or if he feels that the fee is not too high but the combination of fee and frequency is too much for his budget, or if he even angers the psychiatrist by coming to the conclusion that the psychiatrist may not be competent or may not be helpful, the psychiatrist by writing an unfavorable report to the court will succeed in sending the patient to jail. With the therapist in the position of being able to decide on freedom or imprisonment for his patient yet under court order to report to the court at frequent intervals, the development of a normal doctor-patient relationship would be impeded and the freedom of expression required of the patient in psychoanalytically oriented therapy, where he should express whatever he feels or thinks in an uncensored fashion without fear of reprisal, would seem impossible.

6. *The consideration of the Barr-Walker Act as alternative to G's commitment to the state hospital.*

This act, hailed as enlightened legislation when it was passed and still cited as an example of the cooperation of psychiatrist and legislator, will be discussed in greater detail later in this chapter. It applies only to habitual sex offenders; whether it should have been considered in this case seems doubtful.

7. *The Judge's remark about the girls molested: they "will get over it."*

The same remark might be made of every victim of sexual offenses. People do get over these traumatic events in most cases more or less successfully. But the law has never excused criminal actions on the theory that damage has been only psychiatric and not physical and permanent. The whole developing concept of traumatic neurosis is based on the firmly grounded legal concept that emotional traumas are as real as physical traumas.

Psychiatrists who receive responsibility for patients given a psychiatric probation have as much power over them as masters had over indentured servants. For the period of the probation, the psychiatrist's power is almost absolute, subject only to the court's perusal of the reports that the psychiatrist himself furnishes. For this reason, many reputable psychiatrists will not accept a case on this basis, feeling that the inequality in the doctor-patient relationship is inconsistent with the values and principles of psychotherapy. Courts often have not sought out advanced psychiatric opinion on this controversial subject; they are willing to accept the uncontested statements of the "Dr. Fixits" that psychotherapy under these circumstances can be well conducted and has a good prognosis.

Besides psychiatric probation, two other types of disposition made of sex offenders bring them under the authority of the psychiatrist. They are sometimes committed to a state hospital rather than sent to prison, and sometimes sent to prison under special legislation that gives them a status different from that of other prisoners and requires psychiatric examination or treatment. Whether the sexual psychopath statute provides for hospitalization or special type of imprisonment, it has been criticized, in some quarters as too narrow, in others as too broad.[4]

Those who criticize the statutes as being too narrow point out that most criminals and most crimes appear to have some sexual component, even when the crime is not of the kind that is ordinarily considered sexual. "Acts such as stabbing, murders, robberies and arson are sometimes committed as a substitute for the sexual act and consciously or not for the purpose of sexual thrill and excitement." Pennsylvania's Greenstein Act, since repealed, as early as 1933 gave the trial judge power to provide for a mental examination of any convicted criminal who, if found not criminally insane but mentally ill or mentally deficient, could be hospitalized rather than imprisoned. The Maryland Defective Delinquent statute and a similar statute in Connecticut provide that individuals who are either intellectually deficient or emotionally unbalanced, so as to demonstrate clearly an actual danger to society and thereby to require confinement and treatment may be hospitalized rather than sent to prison. The Maryland statute, for example, applies to criminals guilty of a sexual crime, a felony, a misdemeanor punishable by imprisonment in a penitentiary, a crime of violence, or two or more convictions for any offense punishable by imprisonment.[5] Most so-called sexual psychopath laws, however, apply to only those accused or convicted of more clearly sexual crimes.

The sexual psychopath laws have also been criticized as being too broad.

Most sex deviate laws fail to distinguish between the dangerous and non-dangerous sex deviate. The same procedure and possible life confinement is equally applicable to both misdemeanors and felonies. Many sex offenders are mere nuisances and are not dangerous to the safety of society. It is generally concluded that such laws should apply only to conduct involving force or substantial age disparity between the offender and his victim.[6]

Guttmacher and Weihofen have asserted that the sexual psychopath acts are defective because they engraft into the law widely held misconceptions, that sex offenders: can be treated as a homogeneous group of criminals; regularly progress from minor to major sex crimes; and are recidivists, likely to repeat their criminal actions. Curran presents some of the answers given to these arguments. "The claim that it is a misconception that sex offenders regularly progress from lesser to greater crimes may well be correct. However, there are many cases in the criminal courts of defendants who have committed both minor and major sex crimes." Concerning the tendency to recidivism, he points out that there is evidence that sexual criminals do tend to repeat their crimes. "Most psychiatric and psychoanalytic literature indicates that character disorders and neurotic illnesses in this area usually carry with them a high level of repetitive conduct."[7]

The concept of giving help to those with emotional problems that impel them to commit sexual crimes has been enlarged, so that in some states, persons accused of sexual crimes but not yet tried can be committed to state hospitals for treatment. The jurisdictions with "preconviction" statutes are Illinois, Indiana, Iowa, Michigan, Missouri, New Hampshire, Washington, and the District of Columbia. With the exception of Iowa, all these statutes were enacted before 1950; the trend in recent years has been for sexual psychopathy legislation to apply only to convicted sexual criminals.[8]

Birnbaum, in the *New England Journal of Medicine*, has described a case under the Michigan preconviction statute.[9] The defendant, Maddox, in 1952 was alleged to have committed certain sex offenses. He denied these charges. The case never came to trial because in a civil commitment, held prior to trial under the Michigan statute, he was declared to be a criminal sex psychopath and was committed to a state hospital. In the hospital, the defendant continued to deny that he had committed the offenses and the staff therefore felt that he was inaccessible to therapy and recommended that he be transferred to a state prison. Four psychiatrists appeared at this hearing in 1952 to testify against him and to recommend the transfer to prison.

They all went on to testify that incarceration in a state prison and the restraint imposed thereby was, in and of itself, a form of treatment. They claimed that this form of treatment, at least on some occasions, helped to make obdurate sex psychopaths admit their guilt. Thereby, it made them more amenable to the therapy available at the state hospital to which they were returned after they had admitted the commission of the sex offenses. On Maddox's behalf, there was no testimony offered by any psychiatrist to contradict the testimony of the four psychiatrists who testified for the state. Accordingly, for the purposes of this decision, the Court accepted the psychiatrists' testimony without question.

While Maddox was in the state prison, he was treated the same as any other prisoner. He lived, ate and worked just as the other prisoners did. The only difference was that he received a statutorily required interview from a state hospital psychiatrist every six months.

After the hearing, the lower court decided in favor of the state and against Maddox. It is said that Maddox "is getting treatment and the petitioner is properly being confined in . . . prison."

The case was appealed to the Supreme Court of Michigan. In 1958, six years after Maddox had been transferred from the state hospital to prison, the court held that he was improperly held in prison; this ruling did not free him, however, since he was still subject to hospitalization as a criminal sex psychopath. The court did declare itself on the subject of prison incarceration for "treatment" purposes of persons accused but not convicted of crimes:

. . . the Supreme Court of Michigan reversed the lower court's decision and ordered Maddox to be returned to the state hospital or to be released. In its opinion, the Court noted that "the hard fact . . . shows that a person committed under remedial and corrective legislation for hospitalization is, in fact, serving potentially a life sentence in our biggest state prison treated in all respects similarly to other criminals therein confined." The Court also commented that "incarceration in a penitentiary designed and used for the confinement of convicted criminals is not a prescription available upon medical diagnosis and order to any administrative branch of government. Such confinement can only be ordered by a duly constituted court after trial conducted in accordance with the guaranties pertaining to individual liberty contained in the Constitution of this State and this nation. . . . This prisoner has been denied the due process pertaining to criminal trial to which he was entitled before penitentiary sentence or confinement."

Although defendants found to be sexual psychopaths in the preconviction jurisdictions by this reasoning cannot be imprisoned, their stay in a state mental hospital for an indeterminate period, with little chance of definitive therapy or any real treatment at all, may seem not too different from imprisonment. Only three of the preconviction statutes—those of Indiana, Iowa, and Missouri—give the defendant even the right to appeal the finding of psychopathy that is the basis for the hospitalization. Only one of the states with preconviction statutes —Iowa—provides for a court-appointed counsel if the defendant in the psychopathy proceeding is unable to provide his own counsel. And of the eight jurisdictions with these statutes—which, when they were passed, were hailed as enlightened legislation—only four give the defendant the right to a jury determination of his psychopathy. Missouri provides that the use of a jury is discretionary with the judge; Indiana and New Hampshire specifically deny the defendant the right to a jury determination; the Minnesota statute does not deal with the question.[10]

The "postconviction statutes"—found in Alabama, California, Indiana, Kansas, Massachusetts, Michigan, Nebraska, New Jersey, Ohio, Oregon, Pennsylvania, Tennessee, Utah, Vermont, Virginia, Washington, Wisconsin, Wyoming and the District of Columbia—provide that after a normal criminal trial and a conviction, the judge can order, either before he sentences the prisoner in some jurisdictions or after sentencing in others, a psychiatric examination and a determination if criminal psychopathy, according to the definition in the jurisdiction's statute, exists.[11] If so, the prisoner is committed either to a state hospital for treatment in lieu of a prison sentence, or to prison under a special procedure, which usually involves an indeterminate sentence and the recommendation or order of the court that he receive treatment while in prison.

The sexual psychopath who goes to either a hospital or a prison under these statutes in most states does not know how long he will remain held against his will. Unlike the prisoner with a maximum sentence provided by law (with time off for good behavior), the sexual psychopath is almost always held for an indeterminate time. Theoretically, he is to be held until he is cured and no longer a potential danger to society; since these cases are considered among the most difficult to treat and with the poorest prognoses of all those a psychiatrist is called on to treat, the indeterminate sentence usually stretches on for years and, often, for life. Many of these statutes are couched in such terms as the Colorado statute, which provides for a minimum of one day and a maximum of the natural life of the psychopath. Often by statute the psychopath is to be held until, in the words of the Alabama statute, he is fully and permanently recovered.

Only three states provide for a maximum period of incarceration. Connecticut provides that the commitment to a mental hospital cannot be longer than the maximum criminal sentence that could have been imposed. Wisconsin provides that detention is not to exceed the period specified in the sentence for the criminal offense unless the department obtains an order from the committing court to continue the person in the control of the department. Utah—less optimistic about the rehabilitation of the psychopath—provides that all such commitments are for life unless the psychopath is paroled or pardoned. In all other jurisdictions that have similar legislation, the length of stay is determined solely by the statement of the psychiatrist in hospital or prison who must report either that the psychopath is cured or that he has improved sufficiently so that he is no longer dangerous to others before the court will release the offender. Often even after release, probation rather than complete discharge is granted.

To complete the story of the lack of legal safeguards that the committed sexual psychopath has under the laws of most states, in some jurisdictions, after being treated for an indeterminate period in a hospital, the accused can still be forced to serve a jail sentence, at the discretion of the court, under the theory that no double jeopardy is involved since the hospital incarceration is therapeutic and not a criminal punishment. Under these circumstances, it is not difficult to see why the psychopath, who according to psychiatric literature has more difficulty in placing trust than the average patient, does not develop the type of relationship with his therapist that appears to be a necessary part of the successful therapeutic process.

The Canadian law on the subject is not very different from American sexual psychopath laws, but it has been applied more sparingly.[12]

In Canada, the power to legislate with respect to criminal offenses is vested in the federal government, not in the ten provinces. The federal government has designated various sexual activities as sex offenses. In addition, the Criminal Code defines what is called the "dangerous sexual offender" as follows:

"Dangerous sexual offender means a person who, by his conduct in any sexual matter, has shown a failure to control his sexual impulses, and who is likely to cause injury, pain or other evil to any person, through failure in the future to control his sexual impulses or is likely to commit a further sexual offense."

In order to invoke the procedure, the accused person must be convicted of one of six named sexual offenses or an attempt to commit one of them. The hearing must include the evidence of at least two psychiatrists. If the court finds that the accused is a dangerous sexual offender, it has the power to impose a sentence of preventive detention, which may mean life imprisonment in a penitentiary.

From information received from the Department of Justice, it appears that twenty-four persons have been sentenced throughout Canada as dangerous sexual offenders in the years 1955 to 1962 inclusive. This is an average of three persons per year in a population of 18,000,000.

In Canada the procedure for preventive detention is used sparingly. It is a reasonable conclusion that unusual punitive measures do not provide a satisfactory answer to the problem of the sexual offender.

With both lawyers and psychiatrists concerned about the value of the sexual psychopath laws and the lacks in them—the lawyer about the lacks of legal safeguards and the psychiatrist about the lacks of treatment facilities for those convicted under such acts—it is hard to understand why these laws continue to be applied. It is easier to understand why the laws were written. They were originally passed as progressive legislation, although some of the motivation behind the passage of such laws may have been "buck-passing"—the desire of the courts and legislature to turn over to the psychiatrist some of society's most difficult problems. Nevertheless, the rationale and to some extent the motivation behind the sexual psychopath laws were the attempt to apply scientific knowledge and psychiatric healing technics to a class of obviously very irrational but not apparently psychotic accused criminals.

In the process of formulating the legislation, legal safeguards were thrown overboard. Slovenko[13] summarizes legal objections to these laws. "It is objected that due process and equal protection of the laws are denied, especially the right to counsel, to jury trial and to appeal. Other denials or infringements include the rights against self-incrimination and the rights of notice of hearing, personal attendance, subpoenaing of witnesses and cross-examination." In addition to all the legal objections to these laws, the overwhelming practical objection remains—very few psychopaths sent to hospitals or jails under them receive any considerable amount of psychiatric treatment. Like characters in a Kafka novel, they are sentenced to hospital or jail until cured, in a world where none can agree on the definition of "cure" and few wish to attempt to treat it.

A psychiatrist who served as a consultant for a state prison describes the case of an elderly prisoner who was serving an indeterminate sentence for a homosexual offense committed with his eight-year-old nephew. He had previously served a prison term for the same type of homosexual offense and had been on parole. Part of his parole plan was that he was to live with a married sister. Neither the sister nor the parole officer seems to have thought it notable that as part of the parole plan arrangements because of space limitations in the sister's home, the paroled sexual offender and his nephew had to share the same double bed. When the sister learned that her brother had resumed his homosexual practices, she had him rearrested, and now he was sent to jail as a psychopath under a sexual psychopath statute that required that every six months he be reexamined by a psychiatrist to find out whether his condition remained unimproved. He received no treatment at the prison, partly because he would not declare that homosexuality should be considered criminal. Since he apparently had no motivation to change, the two prison psychologists, who had a prison population of thousands to draw on as treatment prospects, preferred to deal with prisoners less argumentative or better motivated.

Every six months, in accordance with the law, the prisoner would receive his psychiatric interview—usually condensed into ten minutes by dictate of the tight schedule of the psychiatric consultant. Every interview, the prisoner was asked if he would resume his homosexual practices if he left jail. If the prisoner had been willing to lie, he undoubtedly would have been given a favorable psychiatric report after the fifteenth or twentieth of these semiannual interviews. Instead, he invariably entered into a philosophic discussion of homosexuality throughout the ages, its popularity in ancient Greece, the findings of the Kinsey report, and other information that seemed to him pertinent. When he was told bluntly that the prison had no real facilities for treating him and that there was no real purpose in his continued stay except that the staff might be subject to criticism if he were allowed to leave in such a frame of mind, he replied, like Luther, that he had taken this course and could take no other. When last heard from, he was still in jail.

The same psychiatrist tells of wanting to write a favorable report on another patient, who appeared to be a good prospect for life outside the prison despite his having received no treatment in the prison. He was told by a prison staff member that because the inmate had been in the prison only a few years, it would look premature to advise his release on the ground that he had been rehabilitated. Several semi-annual examinations later, and after the prisoner had deteriorated dramatically as a result of chronic physical disease, it seemed more appropriate to the prison staff that he be given a favorable psychiatric report; so he was declared to be no longer psychopathic.

Only a few states have received much approbation for psychiatric treatment of sexual offenders.

The 'California Medical Facility' has as its primary purpose the confinement, treatment and care of males under the custody of the Department of Corrections who are mentally abnormal, including psychopathic offenders. The Medical Facility is a prison to the extent that the patients are prisoners serving sentences prescribed by courts, but it differs from the usual prison in that special emphasis is given to the investigation of psychological mechanisms underlying adverse attitudes and conduct. There is a special outpatient clinic for released prisoners.[14]

On the other hand, Bowman and Engle, who are especially familiar with California's institutions and methods, say that "the sex psychopath law is a failure even in California."[15]

Another jurisdiction where major efforts are being made to rehabilitate emotionally unbalanced prisoners including psychopaths is Maryland.

The Patuxent Institution in Maryland has as its aims the treatment and rehabilitation of convicted offenders. Prisoners convicted of a felony, and prisoners who have had 2 or more convictions punishable by imprisonment are eligible for psychiatric examination to determine their suitability for admission. The examination may be requested at any time after conviction and sentence. Insane persons are not accepted. In order to qualify for admission, the offender must suffer from 'emotional unbalance' and must have shown persistent anti-social or criminal behavior. The director of the 400-bed institution is a psychiatrist and the professional staff includes psychiatrists, psychologists and social workers.[16]

In some ways, the fate of a criminal in a prison may be superior to that of an adjudged psychopath in a hospital. For this reason, "when an individual transgresses the criminal code, he has a right to be treated as a criminal."[17] The rights of a criminal are better defined and receive more attention from the law than the rights of hospitalized mental patients and adjudged psychopaths.

Society does not treat sexual psychopaths as criminals but rather as mentally disabled persons. There can be little doubt that such action materially affects their rights. Beyond the obvious change of sentence, there is a basic change in their institutional rights.

The reforms that have swept our penal institutions from the eighteenth to the twentieth century have left mental institutions substantially untouched. Physical restraints have departed from the prison but are still standard equipment in many mental institutions. The overcrowded conditions alleviated in prisons have remained to plague the mental institution. There is doubt about the legality of sterilizing criminals, but sterilization, lobotomy, and electric shock treatment are permissible for sexual psychopaths. Substantial constitutional questions can be raised about the right of a criminal court to expose a defendant to the possibility of sterilization, lobotomy, and electric shock treatment.

In summary, it is fair to say that, in view of the present state of medical knowledge, the lack of procedural safeguards is a fatal defect in sexual psychopath legislation. . . .

In the strong words of a Michigan report: "We dare not, in the 20th Century, blandly deny our whole legal heritage, unique in a world of oppression and bartered blood, and permit ourselves to be stampeded into the dictates of a neoscience."[18]

Whether psychiatry is a neoscience is perhaps not the question. The heart of the matter appears to be the two stools that the psychopath falls between. He is not considered a criminal to the extent that he gets such procedural safeguards and the protection of a maximum sentence to which criminals are entitled. And he is not considered a mental patient to the extent that he gets adequate treatment for his disease. Falling between two stools, he remains—whether in jail or hospital—until an arbitrary decision is made for his release, and, failing this, he may remain until his death.

JUVENILE OFFENDER

The same arguments that have been made for and against the use of rehabilitation facilities for the sexual criminal have been made concerning the juvenile criminal. Originally, the emphasis on treatment rather than punishment was hailed as a humanitarian advance. Increasingly, those treating juvenile offenders have been impressed by the difficulty in securing real changes in late teenage delinquents, partly because they are at an age when relationships with adults are suspect and partly because their previous experiences make them unusually distrustful of adults. When therapy is successful, there is the problem of the disturbed homes and disturbed neighborhoods to which these juveniles have to return.

Dr. Sol Gordon, chief psychologist at New Jersey's Middlesex County Mental Health Clinic, has said that "reports of successes with delinquents are greatly exaggerated. You never read of 'unsuccesses'."

He told a Federal Bar Association panel that in a group of ten boys he had tried to rehabilitate, all were in trouble again within two years, and that no journal was interested in publishing these poor results "because you cannot publish failures in this field." He categorized as a "myth" the claim that more child guidance clinics and more rehabilitation clinics will solve the problem of delinquency.[19]

Others have similarly reported poor results in the treatment of "aimless and indifferent" juvenile subjects who were defendants before the Court of Special Sessions in New York City in 1955 to 56.[20] Twenty-five juveniles who met specific criteria were chosen for this program: they had been charged with a nonsexual offense against persons or an offense against property; they were of average intelligence or better and were not psychotic; they came from homes that were essentially intact; they would cooperate in psychiatric treatment sessions in a court psychiatrist's private office; their mothers and to some extent their fathers were willing to agree to participate in psychiatric casework sessions and submit to psychological tests. These showed the subjects characterized by absence of goals, by lack of pleasure, empathy and loyalty, and by an unremitting mood of boredom. Their delinquent acts (on the average they had committed three known offenses) lacked discernible motivation, real or symbolic: "they robbed when they did not need money, and they assaulted people senselessly and without provocation."

In spite of all the positive factors for therapy, at the conclusion of the study there was "scant, if any evidence of improvement in the subjects. Almost all continued in their goalless behavior and transgressions." The authors suggest that family therapy might have produced equally meager results, but that possibly preschool recognition of "delinquency-prone" children and the establishment of preschool programs of training and emotional enrichment might have been more helpful.

The juvenile, like the sexual psychopath, will not invariably gain from the ministrations of the psychiatrist; like the psychopath, he will suffer from the lack of due process, as the result of the special treatment before the law designed to facilitate his definitive treatment.

The criticism of many lawyers and judges is that juvenile courts are "protecting" delinquents "right out of their basic constitutional rights."[21]

Because juvenile proceedings are said to be "noncriminal," delinquents in many states have been regularly deprived of bail, lawyers, juries, the right to exclude hearsay evidence, and the right to public trial.

Errant children cannot be committed as juvenile delinquents beyond the age of 21. Yet they can be held for weeks or months without a hearing. According to Washington, DC's Judge Orman Ketcham, US county jails hold as many as 100,000 children per year. Moreover, because they can be held to 21, juveniles often get longer sentences than adults do for the same offense.

When appointed in 1957, Judge Ketcham was the sole judge for 225,000 juvenile cases plus all paternity and nonsupport suits, in contrast to the 31 other judges who handled the District of Columbia's 550,000 adult cases. Judge Ketcham has said that he had to hear 197 cases during his first three days of court. He advocates in particular the use of defense lawyers in juvenile courts. In the country's 75 largest cities, less than 10% of juvenile offenders are represented by lawyers. In New York, a new statute will require legal counsel for juveniles, and California has an extensive new statute requiring that juveniles be fully informed of the charges against them and immediately released to their parents unless detention is of urgent necessity. Juveniles are entitled to lawyers by this statute and also required to have them if the misconduct charged is equal to an adult felony.

Lois G. Forer, former Deputy Attorney General of Pennsylvania, has documented some of the charges against the juvenile court process in an article called "Is Juvenile Court Unjust to Children?"[22]

Hundreds of innocent children are in jail in Philadelphia. They were put there unjustly by Juvenile Court.

These boys and girls are suffering this injustice because judges send children to institutions in assembly-line fashion without counsel and without the youngsters even knowing the charges against them. . . .

Some 50 years ago social workers, wishing to mitigate the severity of the criminal law in its application to children, devised Juvenile Court. A wise, compassionate judge, aided by extensive social work, was supposed to reason with the errant child, examine his environment and provide treatment rather than punishment.

The theory was that the child should not be handled as a criminal and, because of that, had no need for the protection of the law. Juvenile Court would act as his parent. . . .

The dream was shattered by social changes. Over-crowding of our city, migration of illiterate people to this area, disruption of families, unemployment and the Negro "revolution" have changed the world we live in.

The way Juvenile Court works now, a boy or mob of boys is brought in for "trial." The arresting officers tell their stories. If the accused is on probation, a probation officer gives his report, which might be mostly hearsay. A school record is read. Then the judge speaks. He doesn't ask the defendant *if* he committed a crime. If the reports are against the youngster, the judge "puts him away."

Every day from 50 to 100 children are being "tried" in Juvenile Court without benefit of counsel. Most of these children are extremely poor and nonwhite.

Many of them—some may be only eight or nine years old—are committed to such institutions as the Youth Development Center, Pennypack House, Glen

Mills, the State Correctional Institution at Camp Hill, Sleighton Farm, St. Gabriel's Hall and other places.

They may remain there until they reach 21. . . .

Two sociologists from the University of California have made similar charges about the standards of juvenile justice after a study of police encounters with juveniles in an unnamed industrial city. The more the youth was apparently respectful of authority, particularly if he were white, the more likely he would be charged with the least offense or let off with a reprimand. "The police officers take what they believe is a clinical attitude towards juveniles; they give more weight to personal character than to actual offense. . . . Such clinical-type decisions are not restrained by mechanisms comparable to the principles of due process."[23]

Although the problems of the sexual psychopath and the juvenile delinquent are not comparable, they can be viewed together from the point of the judicial process because a similar philosophy of detention and treatment has arisen: the accused has been considered a "quasi criminal" rather than a criminal and many of his procedural safeguards have been scrapped in the interests of a presumably more effective or humane treatment. In both cases, the hopes of the innovators who devised these departures from traditional procedures have been largely disappointed. But despite obvious malfunctioning of the judicial process in these areas, and despite well-documented charges, often as sensational as those brought by Forer, the problem remains, possibly because it is so large and so complex that other solutions are not apparent, possibly because of the apathy that prevails when defendants are not in a position to fight for their own rights.

The late Justice Frankfurter was once taken to task for "taking law awfully seriously." His reply was, "I do take law very seriously, because fragile as reason is, and limited as law is as the expression of the institutionalized medium of reason, that's all we have standing between us and the tyranny of mere will and the cruelty of unbridled, undisciplined feeling."[24] In two areas where law has been pushed aside to make way for sociologic or psychiatric progress, the result has been possibly the tyranny of mere will.

CHAPTER 16

Drugs and Addiction

WHEN A MAN takes a drug—whether medication, alcohol or narcotic, whether harmful or harmless—the reasons for his drug-taking may be found in his history, and the effects of his drug-taking will be part of the not completely predictable future. When the drug is as harmless as aspirin is most of the time, or as medically sound as antibiotics are some of the time, the question of the rational basis for the drug-taking does not arise. If a patient has a headache and takes aspirin, or has a bacterial infection and takes an appropriate antibiotic, we can understand the reason for taking medication and we can predict that he probably will recover.

When a drug—alcohol, narcotics, sometimes amphetamines, or hallucinogens like LSD (lysergic acid diethylamide), mescaline or psilocybin—produces irrationality in the taker, or when the need to take a drug is irrational, as in the case of a drug dependence or addiction, we begin to consider controlling either the traffic in the drug or the person who resorts to the drug. Now we are involved in legislation and legislative hearings. Once again the lawyer looks to the physician for some understanding about why the drug was taken and how the taker can be persuaded to take no more; and once again the legislator asks the physician to predict the future, to tell under what conditions or what treatment the drug-taker will be able to resume a place in normal society.

Not all addictions require legislation. A man can become addicted to his wife or his pipe, often to his cigarettes; "the core of the addictive process exists in all of us in such benign forms as cravings for food, tobacco, candy, or coffee. . . ."[1]

Patients have become addicted to placebos even with the knowledge that the placebo was inert and had no medicinal or mood-alleviating effect; the satisfaction that sometimes is derived from possessing a pill and swallowing it can counteract rationality, which states that the pill is not medicinally potent. The law does not deal with these addictions, and psychiatry usually finds them too ubiquitous to deserve treatment, although they interest psychoanalysts studying oral fixations, early influences, and the content of fantasy.

When the addiction is to something that becomes detrimental with continued use or overuse—like reliance on sleeping pills, amphetamines, or narcotics—the need for control of the drug and sometimes the need to treat the drug-taker involve the interest of doctor, lawyer, and legislator.

Claims have been made, in the past, that many drugs expand human consciousness or make available new mental experiences. Cocaine, for example, produces visual and auditory hallucinations, and marihuana (Indian hemp) mood and perceptual changes, without the development of tolerance or withdrawal symptoms. At present much research and experimentation is going on with drugs that have not been shown to be addicting but that do have major effects on consciousness —drugs like LSD, mescaline, and psilocybin. Many of these agents have become known to medicine only in recent years, and psychiatry and the law have not yet determined individually or jointly how dangerous they are and how much control is needed over their use.

DRUGS AS MEDICINE

No one knows the long-range effects of most of the medicines that doctors freely prescribe and patients liberally down, with or against the advice of the doctor. Consider the case of *Johnson* vs *Primm*.[2]

Mrs. Johnson went to her doctor, in 1960, complaining of pains in her back. He prescribed Equanil (pharmacologically known as meprobamate and identical in formula to the product put out by another company as Miltown), a mild muscle relaxant and tranquilizer. The druggist, following directions, dispensed 24 tablets with the instructions that they were to be taken one after meals. A month later, Mrs. Johnson sought to have the prescription refilled; the druggist was told in substance by the doctor that she could "have a few as long as she needs them." Mrs. Johnson took the pills at the rate of 7 to 10 a day for two years, buying them from the druggist in lots of 100 tablets, and then was hospitalized for treatment of meprobamate addiction. During the withdrawal period, she suffered convulsions for six hours, and at that time the diagnosis was made of brain and liver damage caused by the prolonged overdose of Equanil.

The patient and her husband sued the druggist, on the theory that he had failed to exercise due care by selling a drug in excess of the amount prescribed. The druggist successfully defended the suit on the basis of Mrs. Johnson's contributory negligence, and Mrs. Johnson and her husband appealed. On appeal, the New Mexico Supreme Court referred to a physician's affidavit in the proceedings of the trial court, which stated that Equanil tends to destroy the power to resist and is habit-forming when taken in quantity, and sent the case back to the lower court for renewed consideration.

How many Mrs. Johnsons do we have around us? A story considered not sufficiently important to deserve more than the bottom of page 30 of *The Philadelphia Inquirer* of October 29, 1965, gives an indication of the answer. The headline is "Excessive Drug Use Disclosed in Autopsies"; the story concerns a speech by Philadelphia's Medical Examiner to a psychiatric group and his additional remarks to the newspaper's reporter.[3]

Nearly a fourth of the persons examined postmortem by the Medical Examiner's Office last year had "excessive amounts" of drugs in their bodies, Medical Examiner Joseph W. Spelman said Thursday night.

Dr. Spelman said the abuse of drugs—"and I'm not talking about the illegal use of narcotics"—has become an "increasingly alarming problem, particularly in conjunction with alcoholism."

In an interview, Dr. Spelman said evidence of excessive drugs was found in 1,345 cases out of a total of 6,000.

"This does not mean that this many people died of an overdose of drugs," he emphasized. "They died of many things."

"What it does mean is that there were drugs present in the body well in excess of those required for medical treatment."

In about 300 cases, the drugs included excessive amounts of alcohol, he said. About 200 other persons had "huge amounts" of aspirin, and the rest had excessive amounts of barbiturates, tranquilizers and miscellaneous drugs, Dr. Spelman said.

"I don't know if it's a sign of the times, or exactly what it is," the medical examiner said. "But there definitely seems to be a growing tendency for people to be 'hooked' on these barbiturates and tranquilizers."

The progress of the addict as portrayed by a modern Hogarth would begin with glue sniffing in childhood, progress to amphetamines and barbiturates, and culminate in heroin or cocaine. Taking cognizance of the problem, Congress in 1965 passed the Drug Abuse Control Amendments to the Federal Food, Drug and Cosmetic Act, which requires more careful record-keeping along the chain of manufacture and distribution of stimulant, depressant and "psychotoxic" drugs. The issue of "dangerous drugs" had been presented to Congress fifteen years previously, but the policy of the government and Congress during most of this period had been to delay, perhaps on the theory that problems should be allowed to get out of hand before they are tackled. In the intervening years, the illegal and legal distribution of "dangerous drugs" had grown into "grand proportions," with an estimated one-half of the nine billion amphetamine and barbiturate pills produced annually (a pill a week for every man, woman and child in the country) being diverted into illegal channels. In 1964, the President's Advisory Committee on Narcotics and Drug Abuse issued its report stating, what was obvious, that the controls on these drugs were inadequate, and in 1965 President Johnson forcefully recommended enactment of drug control legislation in his messages to Congress both on health and on crime.

A similar bill had passed the Senate in 1964, but passage in the House of Representatives was held up because it was too late in the session to hold adequate hearings. When the earlier bill was debated, the controversial question was whether tranquilizers should be subject to the new controls in the same manner as depressants and stimulants. (The bills did not cover so-called "hard narcotics," including marihuana, which are dealt with by not the Food and Drug Administration but the Narcotics Bureau of the Treasury Department.) In 1965, Congress made it clear that tranquilizers were a major part of the problem and that they would be subject to control, relying on such testimony as that of the then Food and Drug Commissioner George Larrick: "tranquilizers are being increasingly implicated by medical evidence as agents of drug abuse." An FDA staff memorandum had said: "We believe that sufficient evidence has been presented to show that some tranquilizers, like barbiturates, can cause tolerance and psychic and physical dependence."[4]

The new law requires that wholesalers of depressant and stimulant drugs be registered, that inventories and records be maintained so that FDA inspectors can check for illegal diversion, that pharmacists and those physicians who dispense drugs keep prescriptions and invoices for three years, and that prescriptions for specified drugs remain in effect no longer than six months and be refillable not oftener than five times. For the first time, agents of the FDA will be empowered, like the agents of the Bureau of Narcotics, to carry firearms when engaged in undercover operations.

Smuggled drugs from Mexico and other sources will continue to be a problem, but this legislation is the belated recognition of the scope of drug overuse and abuse. That this legislation possibly might not be sufficient to regulate "psychotoxic" drugs was noted by the House Commerce Committee in its report:

The committee was told during the hearings several times that it was unlikely that the enactment of the bill would wipe out the problem in the United States. The committee hopes that the enactment of the bill, plus the institution of voluntary self-regulation on the part of all levels of the drug manufacturing and distributing industries involved, plus increased vigilance on the part of those responsible for prevention of smuggling, will reduce this problem to a minimum and thereby eliminate the possible necessity for the future enactment of more stringent legislation than the reported bill.

The question remains, as asked by Representative J. J. Pickle of Texas, whether we as a people "have become too pill happy."[5]

The problems of the abuse of drugs that are primarily medicines and not narcotics grows daily. Here are some of its manifestations:

The illegal use of nonnarcotic drugs is increasing "at a fantastic rate" among juveniles and young adults.

The use of these drugs has a direct causal relationship to increased crimes of violence.

The use of these drugs is increasingly prevalent among so-called white-collar youth who have never had prior delinquency or criminal records.

The use of these drugs is increasingly identified as a cause of sexual crime.[6]

The use of these drugs is replacing in many cases the use of hard narcotics such as opium, heroin, and cocaine. They are also used to supplement hard narcotics by "budget-minded" addicts who on successive days will use heroin, cocaine, barbiturates, and LSD-25 and then repeat the cycle; this is done not only to reduce the cost of the drug habit but to avoid developing tolerance and physical dependence on any particular drug.[7]

The drugs are often relied on by college students and others under stress for accomplishment, including truck drivers and presumably occasionally airplane pilots, to provide them with the energy to extra production. A Harvard Medical School study has demonstrated that both amphetamines and secobarbital can impair judgment and points to the important practical considerations because "many people make decisions and engage in potentially dangerous activities—such as driving a car—after taking these drugs."[8]

Amphetamines are often used by athletes, including non-human athletes known as horses, although they have been condemned by all official sport regulatory bodies and by the American Medical Association's Council on Drugs and Committee on the Medical Aspects of Sports.[9]

Psychiatrists have called attention to the fact that use of amphetamines for such purposes as control of appetite in obesity or for energy or extra productivity during periods of stress may culminate in periods of frank psychosis or severe depression. The condition of psychic disorganization may be well advanced before psychiatric help is sought; at the time the patient may show insomnia, anorexia, weight loss, suicide attempts, confusion, depersonalization, delusions, hallucinations. The psychiatrist has the dual task of treating the psychiatric illness and the amphetamine dependence.[10]

For the first time, in 1964 an Australian judge granted a divorce in reliance on a section of Australia's Federal Matrimonial Act giving a judge power to dissolve a marriage if one partner has been habitually intoxicated for not less than two years by taking or using to excess any sedative, stimulating, or narcotic drug.[11] The wife, defendant, was habitually intoxicated through excessive taking of a sedative, obtainable without a physician's prescription.

Besides the sociological and psychological effects of these drugs, there is the unanswered question of long-term indirect toxicity and what this could mean in terms of the complex series of biochemical relationships in the human body. Dr. René Dubois of the Rockefeller Institute —speaking of all new substances and technologic innovations, not just of psychotoxic drugs—has warned that we do not understand the indirect and more subtle effects of new additions to our external and internal environment, and that although scientific knowledge is competent to evaluate acute, direct toxic effects, "little is being done in schools of medicine and public health or in research institutes or government laboratories to develop the kind of knowledge that is needed for evaluating the long-range effects on man of modern ways of life."[12]

ALCOHOL

By means of a complicated formula based on the number of reported deaths yearly from cirrhosis of the liver, Jellinek has estimated the prevalence of alcoholism in 12 countries (England and Wales are grouped together). Considering those in the population 20 years of age and older, he has estimated as alcoholic less than 1% of the adult population of Italy; more than 1% of the populations of England and Wales, Australia, Finland, Norway, Canada, and Denmark; more than 2% of the populations of Switzerland, Sweden, and Chile; more than 4% of the population of the United States; and more than 5% of the population of France. One critic, Popham, while not quarreling with the ranking, believes that the percentages are low. The estimate of 1,100 alcoholics per 100,000 population 20 years and older in England and Wales represented over 40 times the number of ascertained mental defectives. In the United States in 1961, according to Federal Bureau of Investigation figures, arrests for drunkenness and drunken driving amounted to about 40% of all arrests made in areas supplying statistics.[13]

Alcohol is not the cause of alcoholism. This dictum was set forth by Mark Keller in 1958, and it is based on his belief that social and psychological—rather than biochemical and physiological—factors are at the root of the addiction to alcohol. He has also given us a good working definition of alcoholism, based on the same belief: "Alcoholism is a chronic behavioral disorder manifested by repeated drinking of alcoholic beverages in excess of the dietary and social uses of the community and to an extent that interferes with the drinker's health or his social or economic functioning."[14]

The acceptance of such a definition leads to the rejection of the view that alcoholism is a disease, or an allergic response to certain chemical factors in alcohol, or an alteration of body chemistry, perhaps on an enzymatic level, that leads to a need for supplies of alcohol. It places alcoholism in the spectrum of such other behavioral disorders as criminal activity, mental illness, addiction to stimulants or psychotoxic drugs, addiction to narcotics, and other forms of deviant—including sexually deviant—behavior. Says Harriet Mowrer[15]:

> Like other forms of personality disorganization, therefore, alcoholism can only be understood as it performs a function in the attempts at social adjustment of the individual. That the consequences of excessive drinking are such as to be only temporarily satisfying, and therefore represent what from an objective viewpoint is inadequate, is of no importance in the understanding of the behavior. What is important is the fact that for the moment at least this type of response (i.e. alcoholism) is within the range of possibilities set by a pattern of personality, for the achievement of what to him seem to be essential goals.

No one pretends to understand thoroughly the interrelationship of body, mind, chemistry, and social forces that culminate in alcoholism. But psychiatrists, especially dynamic psychiatrists, do see alcoholism as an attempted solution to the problems of drives, particularly when their development has become arrested or partially arrested at the oral stage, and when anxieties develop because of conflicts concerning the drives. They see alcoholism as a defensive effort of the individual to protect against disorganization—perhaps in particular to defend against knowledge of dependency, against fear of close relationships, against perverse sexual desires, which are usually latent and not recognized by the alcoholic, and against threat of loss of ego identity. But all of this is too general and too vague to be helpful pragmatically; its value is that it does offer an alternative hypothesis to other theories of the etiology of alcoholism—allergy, biochemistry, and the like—which offer simplified explanations of alcoholism with little or no regard for psychological, interpersonal, and social factors, and which give value only to chemical treatment.

Chief among the physiologic explanations for alcohol is the allergy theory endorsed by Alcoholics Anonymous. Jones argues that to account for alcoholism on such a basis, it would be necessary to argue that it was an excessive sensitivity to alcohol due to previous experience of it. "It is obvious that this is not a description of what happens in cases of alcohol addiction. Far from leading to hypersensitivity, earlier contact with alcohol leads to greater tolerance. The individual needs more and more in order to achieve given effects. In addition, an allergy leads the subject to avoid the exciting substance, whereas in the case of the alcoholic he becomes addicted to it." [16]

Roger Williams attributes alcoholism to biochemical individuality; this theory has been given the title of the genetotrophic theory.[17] There are special appetites, such as the excessive craving of some children for sweets, and the individual metabolic patterns that may lead to over-indulgence are seen as resulting primarily from hereditary differences. A variant of the metabolic approach sees the cause of alcoholism in endocrine underactivity which, when life situations become painful, is alleviated by the alcohol temporarily; the long-run effect, however, is a vicious cycle, because the artificial overactivity caused by the alcoholic intake leads to eventual depletion, which, in turn, is counteracted by more intake of alcohol. The genetotrophic and other physiogenic theories remain sheer speculation. One critic has pointed out that one fallacy is that studies are based on test results showing endocrine or metabolic peculiarities in confirmed excessive drinkers; "it is as likely that their physical peculiarities are a result of drinking as that they are its cause."[18]

If physiologic explanations are accepted, it follows that the reformed alcoholic cannot ever drink again. Although most alcoholics cannot learn to drink moderately, in recent years some authorities have advanced the theory that absolute abstinence is not the only test of control of alcoholism. E. Mansell Pattison, psychiatrist of the National Institute of Mental Health, deals with the assumption that abstinence is a requirement for treatment and is a proof of the results of treatment:

> Is abstinence a criterion of successful treatment? First, there are several studies of abstinent alcoholics which demonstrate deterioration of overall functioning subsequent to abstinence. Second, abstinence may be maintained at the cost of less effective functioning in other areas of life. Third, there are reports of alcoholics who have been rehabilitated who never did stop drinking during treatment, or only stopped for a short while. And finally, there are reports, including our own work, which demonstrate that there are some addictive alcoholics who return to successful social drinking. This evidence does not support the assumption, and I suggest that abstinence must be considered selectively as a condition of treatment, as a goal of treatment, and as a criterion of successful treatment.[19]

It is dangerous to tell an abstinent former alcoholic that he can drink in moderation; the factors that led to the original drinking problem are usually lying in wait, ready to spring again. On the other hand, the evidence that even a few alcoholics *can* drink in moderation after they are rehabilitated is possibly inconsistent with theories of allergy, genetotrophy and hormonal etiology—or at least indicates that such factors are not the whole story. Then the door is open for treatment along psychotherapeutic lines, for attempts to control the alcoholic by psychiatric commitment, and for the application of psychiatric knowledge concerning early relationships, particularly those of mother-child, and development of ability to control impulses and withstand frustration, as a means of attempting to prevent the development of further alcoholics. Once the biochemical theory is questioned, it is reasonable to believe that psychiatrists and lawyers have a useful place in trying to control the drug and the taker of the drug and in trying to prevent new recruits from entering the category of drug takers.

Prohibition was a strictly legal approach that ignored psychological factors; abandoned nationally, the "noble experiment" is still maintained as a local option in many parts of the country. It has been described as causing the problem to become subterranean and the drinker to become devious. Nor has punishment for drunkenness helped. Fines and prison sentences have helped so little that the literature refers to them as the "revolving door" to the jailhouse; Judge William H. Burnett of Denver has spoken of the "street-jail-court-street revolving door," through which pass each year the 1,000,000 arrested for drunkenness in the United States.[20]

Some lawyers have questioned the concept of criminal responsibility for drunkenness; and if alcoholism is truly a disease, as it has been called by the American Medical Association, then we find ourselves in the position of imprisoning people for illness. A more compelling argument for releasing alcoholics from the legal responsibilities of drinking is that criminal intent is necessary for a crime and possibly the alcoholic does not have the capacity to intend the result of his drinking.[21] Opposing these views are the well-established doctrine of tort law that "one who intentionally or negligently becomes intoxicated is held thereafter to the same standard of conduct as if he were sober,"[22] and the principle of criminal law that if one intentionally or negligently becomes intoxicated he is liable for the criminal consequences that arise from the intoxication. Lord Coke, in 1603, observed that those who voluntarily deprive themselves of their reason, such as the drunkard, should not be heard to claim insanity as a defense in a civil or criminal action; the fact that by their own act they had deprived themselves of reason indeed constituted—according to Coke—an aggravation of the offense.[23] But although the fact of drunkenness does not absolve of crime, it often argues against such factors as premeditation and deliberation, and the crime then is held to be of a lesser degree, in the case of murder second-degree rather than first-degree. "A plea of 'not guilty' can be supported only if there was a diagnosable alcoholic psychosis substantially pre-existing the criminal act."[24]

The question of the commitment of alcoholic patients is also a problem for forensic psychiatry, whether the alcoholic wishes to come into the hospital as a voluntary patient or is forcibly hospitalized by a commitment procedure. *Time* reports on the fate of a voluntary patient[25]:

Determined to do something about his weakness for vodka that had earned him a record of minor brushes with the law, Army Veteran Carl Holm, 28, voluntarily went to a veterans mental hospital in Sheridan, Wyo. When he was given town privileges, though, Holm wasted no time getting drunk and passing out on the hospital lawn. "It's my opinion," said a harried doctor after locking up the patient, "that you're a hopeless alcoholic and should spend the rest of your life in this ward."

The hospital duly went to court to ask Holm's involuntary commitment under a Wyoming law that aims to make such hearings easy on the patient. Like similar laws in a dozen other states, Wyoming's is based on a federally sponsored model code. To keep things informal, the code ironically says that a commitment hearing "shall not be bound by the rules of evidence"—the rules that bar hearsay or irrelevant testimony in any ordinary law court.

After a jury ordered Holm back into the hospital last year, his young court-appointed Sheridan lawyer, James E. Birchby, appealed to the Wyoming Supreme Court on the grounds that the jury had been given hearsay evidence about Holm's mental condition. The law permitting this, he argued, denied the due process guaranteed by the 14th Amendment as well as the Wyoming constitution. Last month the court agreed and set Holm free. "It still remains the fundamental law of the land," said the court, "that a person cannot be deprived of his liberty—whether by involuntary hospitalization or some other kind of incarceration—without due process of law."

If hearsay evidence had not been presented, the involuntary commitment presumably would have stood. The catch in voluntary hospitalization procedures is that voluntary commitments can be turned easily into involuntary commitments under the machinery set forth in the statutes of most jurisdictions. In most states that authorize voluntary admissions—of alcoholics or any other class of patient—the patient who has requested admission may be detained in the hospital for a certain fixed period, ranging from two days in one jurisdiction to more than two weeks in others, so that involuntary proceedings may be commenced against him. Even after this fixed period has elapsed, the patient is not necessarily freed; the hospital may further postpone release while it seeks compulsory indeterminate hospitalization.[26] It is easy to see why voluntary hospitalization can be viewed with suspicion by the alcoholic patient.

Many states provide voluntary admission procedures for alcoholics and drug addicts. "The admission procedures for these groups, in most instances, are either identical with or similar to those applicable to the mentally ill."[27]

The Report of the American Bar Foundation states that alcoholics constitute only 1% of patients in mental hospitals.

The current arguments in favor of a wider use of the hospitalization provisions for alcoholics will thus have to be reviewed in the light of the additional burden that such an influx of patients would place on the existing facilities. Moreover, experience with the compulsory hospitalization of such patients leads one to question the efficacy of such an approach to the treatment of alcoholism.[28]

However, New York, which has admitted alcoholics to state hospitals on a voluntary basis since 1961, when the Department of Mental Hygiene established special alcoholism units in two institutions, recently passed a law providing for involuntary admission on the certificate of two physicians.[29]

Perhaps the dilemma that law and psychiatry find themselves in when dealing with the alcoholic can be simply summed up. Under a truly voluntary type of hospitalization, the typical alcoholic will not wish to remain in a hospital long; one of the character problems of alcoholics is their superficiality when dealing with their disease, their denial of its severity and their optimism concerning their ability to deal with the problem on their own. On the other hand, most involuntary commitment procedures apply only to those who are a threat to themselves and to others, and most alcoholics do not constitute such a threat.

An example of the distinction between the treatment of alcoholics and drug addicts, on one hand, and the mentally ill on the other, is found in the Pennsylvania Mental Health Act of 1951. Both alcoholics and drug addicts are included within the single definition of "inebriate." " 'Inebriate' shall mean a person who is so habitually addicted to the use of alcoholic or other intoxicating or narcotic substances as to be unable to stop the excessive use of such substances without help. The term shall include 'dipsomaniac,' 'drug addict,' and 'habitual drunkard'."[30] Inebriates can apply for voluntary admission, like persons thought to be mentally ill, to the superintendent of any mental hospital, but they can in addition also apply for admission to an institution for the care of inebriates or a general hospital maintaining a psychiatric department or ward. But medical commitments are not allowed to inebriates, although they are valid for the mentally ill, mental defectives, and epileptics. The emergency detention procedure applies only to the mentally ill and not to inebriates or other categories of patients. The court commitment, an alternative to the medical commitment under Pennsylvania law in the case of involuntary patients, is used for only a minority of the mentally ill; however, it must be used for the involuntary commitment of an inebriate. The petition to the court need be by any responsible person in the case of the mentally ill who is dangerous to himself, by a guardian, relative or friend in the case of a person who is thought to be mentally ill and in need of observation, diagnosis and treatment, and by at least two citizens "who shall be his spouse, parent, child, committee of the estate or next friends" in the case of the inebriates. For inebriates, unlike other categories of inmates, no detention shall be "for a period of more than one year." In such ways has the legislature tried to provide for the hospitalization of the alcoholic, who does not meet the criteria of mental illness, with some safeguarding of civil liberties.[31]

Most alcoholics do not require hospitalization; if they are motivated or influenced to seek or receive treatment, they are seen in doctors' offices, often by the general practitioner and not by a psychiatrist, or by social agencies or ministers doing pastoral counseling, or they become involved in Alcoholics Anonymous or other self-help mutual-help groups. Of the minority of alcoholics who do need hospital treatment, many need relief from symptoms of acute alcoholism, which is a problem of medical management in a general, not a psychiatric hospital. Other severely addicted alcoholics are only secondarily alcoholics; they are primarily schizophrenic or depressive, or fit some other psychiatric category under which they can be hospitalized. If two estimates are correct—that there are 5,000,000 alcoholics in the United States and that only 3% of the resident population of state mental institutions (or about 16,000 patients) carry the diagnosis of alcoholic—then only one out of every 300 alcoholics is in mental hospitals at any one time. In the case of drug addiction, there is a similar disparity between the seriousness and extent of the problem and the number of patients who receive treatment in hospitals. To some extent these disparities may result from the disappointing results of psychiatric treatment for these addictions.

When the proposal was made to Congress that a seven-man federal commission on alcoholism be set up to conduct research on alcoholism, disseminate information, establish hospitals and clinics for alcoholics, and contract with other institutions for the treatment of alcoholics, the American Medical Association opposed the measure on the ground that "the problems of alcoholism can best be solved through cooperative efforts of lay, medical and governmental groups," whose efforts, the Association stated, had obviated the need for such a commission. "The American Medical Association and its Committee on Alcoholism, Alcoholics Anonymous, state and local governments, and the Department of Health, Education, and Welfare, particularly the National Institute of Mental Health and the Division of Community Health Services of the Public Health Service, can be justly proud of their efforts and accomplishments."[32] Other observers see the problem of alcoholism as growing, extending into new groups, such as the older adolescent and the younger housewife, and requiring greater community cooperative effort from social agencies, medicine, psychiatry, rehabilitation and other services.

THE DRINKING DRIVER

A drawback to a career in science, sometimes, is that after a rigorously designed research project gives proof of something that has been merely a hypothesis, a common reaction is that "we knew it all along, anyway." Recent scientifically designed tests have validated a relationship between alcohol ingestion and traffic accidents. The number of traffic fatalities since 1899 having reached the incredible total of almost two million, social scientists during the last decade have begun more seriously to explore the interrelationship of these factors, although common sense had already told us that the relationship of alcohol to auto accidents was deadly real.

But although we have always known of this relationship, and although we are able to validate the relationship with scientific tests that indicate at what levels of blood alcohol impairment of performance begins to be obvious, the answer is not as easy as "if you must drink, don't drive." Psychiatrists are aware, first that alcohol impairs judgment and that in the chronic alcoholic disorders of thinking become prominent. We cannot appeal to the alcoholic on the grounds of reason to the same extent that we can to a "normal" person, because of the physiologic effect of the alcohol on him and perhaps also because of basic flaws in his personality and thinking that may predate the alcohol problem. We cannot tell a drinking driver that discretion is the better part of valor; both the nature of his emotional problem and the effect of the alcohol on his system encourage him to ignore good advice. The drinking-accident relationship "may be as much the result of psychiatric processes associated with pathological drinking as it is of physiologic changes attributable solely to the pharmacologic effect of alcohol."[33]

Second, if we consider not only the warped psychological processes that impair rational thinking but the deeper psychological motives involved in the dynamics of some alcoholics—self-destructiveness, hostility, and the desire to escape from the inhibitions of everyday life— we see the relationship of drinking and driving as potentially extremely pathologic. When Russian roulette is played with a pistol, the pathology is obvious; when the same game is played with an automobile, the pathology is less obvious but affects more people. We cannot estimate the percentage of automobile accidents that result from alcohol plus a desire to die, to risk death, to express deep destructive feelings or perhaps, merely the addicting desire (known to the compulsive gambler, sky-diver, check-passer, stock market plunger) to experience the warm glow of having ascertained that the lovely Lady Luck is still on one's side.

Records of New York City traffic fatalities indicate that possibly we have been underestimating the effect of alcohol on auto deaths. Of all motorists killed there in 1957, 55% had been under the influence of alcohol. The Chairman of the AMA's Committee on Chemical Tests for Intoxication, Dr. Herman Heise, stated in 1958 that if all drinkers, not merely alcoholics, were prevented from driving, the yearly toll of auto deaths could be drastically reduced: "possibly half of our 40,000 people doomed to die on the highways could live, and a half million more could be spared from painful and crippling injuries."[34]

At a meeting of the American Psychiatric Association in 1965, a study was presented of drivers responsible for 72 fatal traffic accidents in Washtenaw County, Michigan, an area including Ann Arbor and the surrounding rural area. Only 13 of the 72 had survived the accidents. Fifty of the accidents—more than two-thirds—involved only the driver's car and no pedestrians. Half occurred between Friday at 6 PM and 6 AM Monday. "Of all the drivers, 29 (40%) were alcoholics and 7 (10%) were prealcoholics. Additional candor on the part of various respondents—or just additional respondents—would have increased the size of the alcoholism group." A significant number of alcoholic drivers had suffered depression, had attempted suicide, or seriously considered it. Some of the men were extremely violent, particularly after drinking; they had histories of recurrent assaults on other persons. The alcoholics and prealcoholics in the group averaged three times the number of previous accidents of the nonalcoholics. The 29 alcoholic drivers had 17 previous convictions for intoxicated driving, whereas the group of seven prealcoholics and the group of 36 nonalcoholics each had only one such conviction. Of the 29 alcoholics, 45% had either a drunk-driving or a drunk-and-disorderly conviction.[35]

It is becoming clear that a substantial number of drinking drivers who precipitate grave traffic accidents are chronic alcoholics. Arrests and penalties for drunk-driving or drunk-and-disorderly offenses do not protect the driving public. Suspending or revoking the driver's license is a dubious gesture; 5 of the 72 drivers were driving without a license at the time they caused a fatality because their license had been previously revoked. One subject came to Michigan from an adjoining state where he had just been released from a state mental hospital after having undergone treatment for habitual alcoholism. He had lost his license as a result of three drunk-driving convictions. He promptly purchased a car and wrecked it a few weeks later while driving in an intoxicated condition. His passenger, a young woman, was killed. The alcoholic driver today, even when repeatedly apprehended, is neither effectively restricted from driving nor required to seek treatment. He continues his depredations until he removes himself by way of a fatal injury. Only a program designed to protect, restrain and rehabilitate the alcoholic driver will protect the public from the "inevitabilities" which are now misnamed "accidents."

What to do about the problem? Experience in Scandinavia has shown that greater concern on the part of society for its own safety and strict enforcement, as expressed in heavy fines, long jail sentences, and less favoritism for the well-to-do as compared to the less affluent, "have made a distinct impact in the Scandinavian countries and, if nothing more, . . . generated a respect for drinking-driver legislation, which is nonexistent in the United States."[36] Contrasting with the Scandinavian program of strict enforcement, in the United States legislation, passed or proposed, dealing with the problem involves greater departures from traditional legal practice.

The blood test has been considered a reliable determination of intoxication. A physician is needed to administer it and to interpret its results in court, and constitutional questions have been raised about the privilege against self-incrimination; should a patient's blood—any more than his own words or the words of his wife—be allowed to determine his guilt? New York in 1953 was the first state to pass a law stating that by operating a motor vehicle on a public highway a driver at the same time gives implied consent to have a blood sample drawn and used as evidence in the event of arrest. The New York law merely clarified existing practice in most state and federal jurisdictions, which had allowed the taking of the blood sample without the consent of the person. Since the passage of the New York law, an additional thirteen states—Connecticut, Iowa, Kansas, Minnesota, Missouri, Nebraska, New Hampshire, North Dakota, Oklahoma, South Dakota, Utah, West Virginia, and Vermont—have passed implied consent laws concerning driving. A typical statute (New Hampshire) provides:

Any person who operates a motor vehicle upon the public highways of this state shall be deemed to have given consent to a chemical test or tests of his blood or urine for the purpose of determining the alcoholic content of his blood, if arrested for any offense arising out of acts alleged to have been committed while the person was driving or in actual physical control of a motor vehicle while under the influence of intoxicating liquor.[37]

The British Medical Association has recommended and the British Minister of Transport supported the introduction of a road-safety bill which would make it an offense to drive a motor vehicle with more than a specified level of alcohol in the blood. The level being considered is 80 mg of alcohol in 100 ml of blood—representing "a consumption of 9 to 12 whiskies." Impetus for these measures was the 1964 record of 119 deaths on the roads in England and Wales over the Christmas holiday period. For a two-month period that included the holidays, tests on 733 people killed on the roads showed that at least 38% of the drivers had been drinking (evidenced by blood alcohol levels of 5 mg per 100 ml), and of this group 75% had levels over 50 mg and 50% had levels over 100 mg, the latter figure representing 12 to 15 single whiskies. The proposed legislation was favored by more than 85% of a sample of drivers interviewed in a national poll. Similar legislation has been proposed in Canada, and the Chairman of the American Medical Association Committee on Automotive Safety has recommended that the "new offense" of driving with a blood level of 0.08% alcohol be adopted in United States jurisdictions. Such legislation "would create a situation comparable to exceeding a 60-mile-per-hour speed limit, failing to yield the right of way, etc. It would not pose any moral issue—as does a charge of inebriation—nor connote incompetence—as would reckless driving charges—and such an offense should be much easier to prosecute and enforce."[38]

The proposal has been made that alcoholism be made a legally reportable disease so that alcoholic drivers can be effectively curbed. "Many physicians may object to this suggestion as inimical to the patient-doctor relationship. However, how many of us would let Typhoid Mary walk out of our office to resume a job as short-order cook at a local restaurant?" The physician would require legal assurance that in reporting alcoholism to a state driver-licensing agency he would be protected from civil suit which might be brought by the patient, and the physician and patient both "must be persuaded that the abrogation of the doctor-patient relationship entailed by such reporting is justified." Those making this proposal point out that the reluctance of doctors to make such disclosures, which lead to patient distrust of doctors, may rule out this possible approach.[39] That many drivers need their licenses to earn their livelihoods makes this an especially threatening area to abrogate confidentiality; psychiatrists in particular feel that confidentiality is a prerequisite for the therapeutic relationship.

The problem of the drinking driver is only a facet of the total problem of the alcoholic in modern society, given particular immediacy by the potential of causing death to innocents who happen to cross his path. The medical and psychiatric answer to the problem includes not only specific proposals for controlling use of the highways but the more general measures needed to rehabilitate a patient usually hard to work with and whose treatment requires cooperation from many sources in the community. A proposed plan for dealing with the total problem of the alcoholic in the District of Columbia, for example, makes the treatment and rehabilitation of the alcoholic an integral part of a comprehensive community mental health plan, calling on the cooperation of psychiatric hospitals, general hospitals, nursing homes, physicians in private practice, Alcoholics Anonymous, churches, missions, departments of vocational rehabilitation and public assistance, and offering to the alcoholic such facilities as outpatient clinics, half-way houses, neighborhood centers, a detoxification unit, a rehabilitation farm, a hostel, and long-term security hospitalization. Chief Judge David L. Bazelon of the United States Court of Appeals for the District of Columbia called this plan "most promising," but pointed out that legal and administrative methods to direct the individual to the appropriate unit for treatment present difficult problems that will have to be solved by a sharing of responsibility by experts in the problem of alcoholism, legislators, and public administrators.[40]

DRUG ADDICTION AND DRUG TRAFFIC

The narcotic-control laws on the federal and state levels in this country provide the severest criminal penalties of any laws with the possible exception of murder. Maximum sentences of forty or more years, as well as an increasing number of life sentences, are the law in many states. Death penalties have been added for sale to minors. Nearly half the states have some limitation on suspension, probation or parole that apply specifically to narcotics offenders.

The aim of these laws—called savage in their application by many legal authorities—is to dry up the source of infection, the illegal traffic in narcotics. When medical authorities object, the law-enforcement authorities retort that this is perfectly good preventive medicine, particularly when methods of treatment for narcotic addicts have not been overly successful. Nevertheless, many legal authorities, along with most medical authorities, have opposed criminal-law enforcement as the *sole* means of attacking the addiction problem.[41]

In *The Addict and the Law*, Lindesmith makes some important distinctions. His concern is with addiction to opiate drugs and their equivalents—opium, opium derivatives such as morphine and heroin, and synthetic opium equivalents such as demerol, methadone, codeine, dilaudid, and percodan—and he emphasizes the relative normality of addicts to these drugs contrasted to the abnormal state of the alcoholic, barbiturate addict, or person under the influence of marihuana or cocaine. "Opiate-type drugs do not directly incite to crime or to irresponsible behavior as alcohol does, for example. They have a sedative, tranquilizing effect and if all other things were held equal would probably inhibit rather than encourage crime. The crimes of drug users are overwhelmingly crimes against property committed to secure the means of obtaining drugs."[42] After the initial use of the drug, the taker becomes dependent and thereafter uses the drug primarily to avoid the unpleasant reaction that occurs when he stops; as long as he takes the drug regularly he appears and seems relatively normal. "It is not possible to determine reliably by casual observation whether a given person is or is not under the influence of heroin."[43]

Marihuana, on the other hand, is not a habit-forming drug; its regular use does not produce tolerance and its abrupt cessation does not lead to withdrawal distress. Its effects are experienced as exhilaration, loss of inhibitions, a changed sense of time and other sensations somewhat comparable to the stimulating effects of alcohol, also an intoxicant. Lindesmith states, however, that marihuana is less dangerous and less harmful to the body than alcohol—it is not associated with medical pathology, such as the cirrhosis of the liver or neuropathies resulting from alcohol. He describes smoking of marihuana as a "minor problem"; "ironically, the accusations that are leveled at marihuana are all applicable to alcohol. . . ."[44]

The extent of the drug addiction problem is unknown. Before the passage of the Harrison Narcotic Act in 1914, drug addiction was a common medical problem; probably the users at that period were on the average older and more affluent than many of today's addicts, and included many women. Addiction was easy to acquire "innocently"; many of the drugs sold without prescriptions, for coughs, "female complaints," "nerves," and what modern advertisers call "tired blood," contained opium derivatives. The popular paregoric was and is a camphorated tincture of opium and Dover's powder a combination of ipecac and opium.

The civilian population had unlimited access to patent medicines such as Perkins Diarrhea Mixture and Mrs. Winslow's Soothing Syrup, whose principal active ingredients were narcotics and for which claims were made that they cured almost all human ills, especially another form of addiction, alcoholism. The well-equipped medicine chest in the Gilded Age almost certainly contained a ball of opium and a bottle of paregoric.[45]

Although addiction tended to begin at a later age than at present, many young children and adolescents were addicts. In 1885 an estimated 1% to 4% of the population was believed to be addicted,[46] or 550,000 to 2,200,000 persons.

The basic antinarcotic statute in the United States, the Harrison Act, was ostensibly a revenue measure; the imposition of an excise tax —with the accompanying requirements of special forms for the transfer of drugs and the requirement of registration for all persons and firms handling drugs—was designed to make the process of drug distribution of public record. Lindesmith has found no indication of any legislative intention to deny addicts access to legal drugs or to interfere with medical practice as it affected the addict. Even veterinary surgeons could continue to dispense drugs to their patients! The Act stated, in clear terms:

Nothing contained in this section shall apply: (a) to the dispensing or distribution of any of the aforesaid drugs to a patient by a physician, dentist, or veterinary surgeon registered under this Act in the course of his professional practice only.[47]

Lindesmith refers to two unusual features of the narcotics control program established under this Act. The program was not established by legislative enactment or by court interpretations of such enactments; the act was ostensibly a revenue act. The narcotics control program was established by administrative decisions of officials of the Treasury Department of the United States. Also, while in legal theory revenue measures, the federal narcotics laws as subsequently amended contain "penalty provisions among the harshest and most inflexible in our legal code."[48]

In 1919, the Supreme Court ruled that a prescription of drugs for an addict to keep him comfortable by maintaining his customary use was not a prescription of drugs within the meaning of the law and did not come within the exemption granted the doctor-patient relationship.[49] As a result, Treasury Department regulations could prevent the physician from providing narcotics for a user "to keep him comfortable by maintaining his customary use. . . ." The obvious result is that addicts have had to turn to nonmedical and illegal sources of drugs to satisfy their craving. In 1922, the *Behrman* case ruled that medical prescriptions for drugs for addicts were illegal despite the fact, stipulated by the prosecution, that the prescriptions were for the purpose of treating and curing addicts; one basis for this decision was that vast quantities of drugs had been prescribed.[50]

These early decisions have been modified by a 1925 case, *Linder* vs *United States*.[51] A physician who had dispensed four tablets to a woman, in fact a police informer, and been convicted under the Harrison Act, was exonerated in his appeal to the Supreme Court. Still the rules, regulations and policies of the Federal Bureau of Narcotics—based on the theory that addiction is not a disease, to be treated with his best judgment by a physician, but a wilful indulgence meriting punishment and separation from medical help—are substantially as they were in 1922 regarding the physician's responsibility for the care of addicts. Under these regulations, regular administration of drugs to addicts was declared to be legal only in the case of aged and infirm addicts in whom withdrawal might cause death, and of persons afflicted with such diseases as incurable cancer.

The penalties provided by law for violations are not only harsh but equally applicable to addict, illegal drug peddler, and the physician who dispenses more drugs than regulation allows. The Harrison Act provided for a maximum term of ten years; the sentencing judge in his discretion could impose a lesser or a suspended sentence. In 1951 the Boggs Bill (the Boggs Amendment) and in 1956 the Narcotic Drug Control Act not only provided for procedural changes that make it easier to secure convictions but prescribed mandatory sentences, leaving the judge no discretion to modify the sentence to the special circumstances of the case. Present penalties—applicable to addict, peddler, physician—provide for sentences of two to ten years, with probation and parole permitted for a first possession offense; mandatory five to 20 years, with probation and parole excluded for second possession or first sale offense; mandatory ten to 40 years, with probation and parole excluded for third possession or second sales and subsequent offenses; and ten years to life, with probation and parole excluded, or a death sentence if recommended by a jury, for sale of heroin by one over 18 to one under 18. Parole has thus been eliminated in all cases except the first conviction for possession; unlike most other federal prisoners who become eligible for parole after serving one-third of their sentences, narcotics offenders must serve two-thirds (narcotics offenders do have the chance to have the final one-third of their sentence forgiven if they earn credit for good behavior in prison.)

The harsh penalties deter doctors from becoming interested in treating addiction. They may deter some peddlers, but most of the penalties are imposed on the addict, who is not easily deterrable.

Following the passage of the Boggs Act in 1951, many states passed "Little Boggs Laws" to increase the penalties in their own jurisdictions. Vetoing the New Jersey bill, Governor Robert Meyner gave some examples "culled, not from a fertile imagination, but from the hard experience of men charged with enforcement of narcotic laws."

Some university students, while at college, acquired marihuana from a peddler and distributed some of it to friends in New Jersey while home on vacation. The students were convicted but sentence was suspended and the defendants placed on probation. These young men have gone on to become useful and valuable citizens. But under Assembly Bill No. 433, they would have to be sentenced to 10 years at hard labor, and if one of the students was 21 years or over and the marihuana was given to one under 18, the mandatory minimum of 20 years would be imperatively imposed.

A druggist who answered an emergency call of a physician and delivered a narcotic without a written prescription would face a mandatory minimum of 10 years, beyond the power to suspend. An inexperienced drug clerk who sold more than 4 ounces of Brown's Mixture or Stokes Expectorant without a prescription would face a mandatory sentence of 10 years, and if the buyer was under 18 and the clerk was over 21, to a mandatory 20 year sentence. A druggist or physician who fails to maintain the detailed records required by chapter 18 or to retain them for the prescribed period would have to be incarcerated for a minimum of 2 to 10 years depending upon which of the many sections of the act he violated because these bills would forbid the suspension of sentence and probation. One who violates the provisions of the act relating to labeling would, without regard to varying circumstances, be subjected to the mandatory minimum of 10 years.[52]

The severity of the sentences mandatorily imposed by federal law and in most states had two very apparent results. Since the power to modify sentences is denied judges, the police and the prosecutors have a potent weapon to influence defendants: by offering to allow the defendants to plead guilty on a lesser charge or by making other "deals," they can fix sentences in many cases. Second, the prosecution of marihuana dealers and users is minimal: since most enforcement authorities do not consider use of this drug comparable to "hard narcotics," the mandatory sentences seem disproportionately long.

The Federal Bureau of Narcotics has found the Harrison Act and the philosophy that has developed around it effective in deterring and controlling the use of narcotic drugs. Harry Anslinger, the controversial former director of the Narcotics Bureau, estimated that the number of addicts was 200,000 in 1914, before the passage of the Harrison Act (a much lower figure than that of some other authorities), or 1 in 400 persons in the United States, that this figure reached a low of 20,000 in 1945, and was between 50,000 and 60,000 in 1955, an incidence of 1 in 3,000 of the population. However, other authorities state that there are as many addicts in New York City now as Anslinger found in the entire country then.[53]

On the basis of the Anslinger statistics, three Public Health Service doctors in *JAMA* in 1948 found the narcotics menace minimal.[54]

When the Harrison Narcotic Act was passed in 1914 there were possibly 150,000 to 200,000 narcotic addicts, mostly women, in the United States. Now . . . there is about 1 addict per 3,000 of population, or a total of approximately 48,000, mostly men. This reduction has been largely due to the vigorous enforcement of the Harrison Narcotic Act and to Federal facilities for the treatment of addicts. Compared with the problem arising from the abuse of drugs such as barbiturates and alcohol, narcotic addiction is not a great public health hazard.

The *JAMA* article so impressed one Chicago newspaper that its news story was headlined, "Find Narcotics Beaten as US Health Menace."[55]

What is the extent of the drug problem? Lindesmith, who has been studying and writing of it since 1935, will not even presume to guess, concluding only[56]

that the number of addicts in the United States in 1914 is unknown and cannot be reliably estimated; that it is even more hazardous to estimate the extent of the problem today; and that federal narcotics officials have, over a long period of years, underreported and underestimated the problem.

In contrast to the American, much attention has been paid to the British system of drug control, which maintains addicts on free narcotics supplied by the Government. Under it, there is said to be little traffic in narcotics, since the user can always obtain them through legitimate channels. In the absence of the narcotics "pusher," fewer addicts are recruited and less financial incentive given to seduce a nonuser into becoming a user.

Addicts in England are sometimes described as "registered" with the government. There is no official registration, but addicts consider themselves registered when they are known to a physician and regularly receive supplies. The Home Office does maintain an index of known addicts, compiled largely from pharmacists' registers. According to the official Home Office index, there were 753 "known addicts" in the United Kingdom in 1964; some authorities believe the total number ten times this figure, but the Home Office feels that there may be, at the most, two or three unknown addicts for each name on the current index.

Some concern has been expressed about the breakdown of the system and an increase in the number of users caused by resale of legally obtained narcotics by "registered" addicts to novitiates. Dr. Thomas Bewley, consulting psychiatrist at Tooting Bec Hospital, London, has recommended compulsory notification when drug addicts become known to a physician. He has also said: "If potential addicts had less contact with addicts and less ease of access to narcotics, there would be less addiction."

The narcotics problem is not only of smaller dimension in Great Britain; it is also more centralized. Almost all known addicts are in London, although the Manchester police have recently appointed a drug squad.

Although the British system has often been praised, a government committee headed by Lord Brain has recommended changes in it that would bring it closer to the American model. It noted that six doctors in Great Britain write a large proportion of the prescriptions for addicts and that some doctors write single prescriptions for 1,000 pills. The Brain Committee, in 1961, had endorsed the system of complete liberty for individual doctors to prescribe drugs in any quantity that they feel fit; its 1965 report, noting increased addiction, recommended that special centers be set up for treating addicts, with power to detain patients compulsorily if they try to leave, and prescribing drugs for addicts except at these centers be outlawed.[57]

The attempt to put the United States on a similar permissive prescribing of narcotics has met with much opposition. Senator Jacob

Javits feels that controversy over the British system—over what the system really is, whether addicts can be maintained on stable dosages, whether chemical substances such as methadone can be utilized, whether conditions in the United States are comparable to those in Britain— diverts us from the task of providing an improved American system now. He is a sponsor of four pending bills in Congress designed to promote a new approach to the addiction problem. Two of the related series of bills would provide Federal aid to state and local governments and nonprofit private groups to provide treatment and rehabilitation programs in or near the home communities of the addict. Senator Javits contrasts the present system with a more desirable approach.[58]

The Federal experience consists of approximately 800 convictions each year; only two Federal Hospitals—at Forth Worth, Texas, and Lexington, Kentucky—deal with the subject, and they register a staggering rate of recidivism. . . . Everyone who has studied the matter agrees that the two existing Federal hospital facilities in their present locations—whatever their intrinsic merit—cannot begin to meet the tremendous need for rehabilitative aftercare, involving a wide range of services—medical, psychiatric, psychological, family counseling, job training—which appear at this point to be the only approach which has a chance of meeting the narcotics challenge.

A third bill would authorize Federal civil commitment for the treatment of narcotics users as an alternative to criminal prosecution and imprisonment. A fourth would ameliorate the rigid restrictions on the postconviction sentencing in the Federal courts of addict defendants. The purpose of the legislative proposals would be to replace punitive measures with rehabilitative, and to give the doctor authority to withdraw drugs from the patient at the rate he feels is best.

The most recent advance in the treatment of addicts has been the substitution of methadone, hailed on the basis of experimental tests as a chemical substance that satisfied the craving for narcotics without providing a euphoric "kick."[59] The work of Dole and Nyswander in treating addicts by this method has received wide publicity, but Vogel has criticized the original study on the grounds that it dealt with too few patients, that those in the series had not been followed for sufficient periods of time, and that the study had not seriously considered the possibility of methadone addiction becoming a problem—as the heroin treatment for morphine addiction and the demerol treatment for heroin addiction became problems.[60]

Perhaps the greatest and the only respectable success rate in cure of addiction is that of San Francisco's Synanon Foundation, a private organization based on principles like those of Alcoholics Anonymous and practicing a kind of leaderless and informal group therapy in a communal living setting. In contrast to the Federal and state hospital records of success with barely one in ten patients, Synanon claims that fully 50% of 1,275 addicts who have participated in its program are off drugs, and that more than 90% of members who completed the full 30-month program have remained abstinent.[61]   Dr. Bernard Casselman, Synanon's Director of Medicine, has opposed the practice of maintenance dose therapy.[62]

I wonder if this agitation for 'free drugs' is motivated by our own dilemma, our own inadequacy in not knowing how to handle this problem. . . . I have never seen alcohol, free or otherwise, as the suggested treatment of alcoholism.

I feel sympathetic toward any diseased individual. I will not potentiate the seriousness of his illness by supplying drugs. Drugs are not the problem, drugs are not wanted by addicts, drugs are not therapeutic for addicts, drugs have been tried before and never worked, drugs will not solve our problems with the addict.

Besides the basic controversy concerning treatment, other questionable areas concerning drugs are:

Differences of opinion concerning whether marihuana, used by musicians, beatniks, collegians, and other groups sometimes characterized by superego deficiencies, is extremely harmful and whether it potentiates criminal behavior.

Differences of opinion concerning treatability of even a minority of addicts as outpatients.

The problem of the addict who commits a crime to secure money to satisfy his addiction and is arrested. In the process of serving a sentence for the crime, he may miss the opportunity for treatment of the addiction.

The same problems of need for commitment to secure treatment and the consequent deprivation of civil liberties that are found with the alcoholic. Part of this problem is that the committed patient does not necessarily receive adequate treatment, even in light of conflicting opinions of what constitutes adequate treatment.

State law has paralleled Federal law in strictness; but in this field there have been two developments. In 1962, in *Robinson* vs *California*,[63] the Supreme Court declared unconstitutional the legislation that in 19 states made drug addiction in and of itself criminal. Since 1961, three states—California, New York, and Massachusetts—have by law provided for rehabilitation systems. Their laws established commitment procedures with required aftercare programs and provided that for certain addicts—those with less serious prior criminal records—commitment and rehabilitation can substitute entirely for a criminal sentence when the addict is under arrest and is tried for a crime. The California rehabilitation program is open to not only confirmed addicts but also persons "in imminent danger of becoming addicted." This criterion, of dubious constitutionality as a ground for civil commitment, has been rejected by the other two states. "These laws are a testament

. . . that even the harshest of the criminal statutes can be modified, and treatment substituted for punishment."[64]

PSYCHEDELIC DRUGS

Among the great adventures of our time is the invasion of the inner space of the mind. Freud stimulated research in mental operations and his theories and clinical data concerning the unconscious processes of the mind revolutionized many previous concepts. Psychoanalysis, with its verbal and intuitive probing of the hidden mind, the interpretation of dreams as a clue to inner needs and desires, and developments in other branches of the behavioral sciences, are revealing far more information about what goes on in our minds than man has ever known before.

While the use of drugs is not new in dulling the conscious and opening up unconscious behavior, fresh developments present fascinating possibilities for further exploration and therapy, but also for danger—both to the individual and to society. Chemical attempts to explore the wonders of the mind are associated with such giants as William James, Aldous Huxley, Gerald Heard and others. The hallucinogenic fungi of Mexico were widely used by Indians long before modern chemistry was known. Today, a brand of mental drugs is on the market—mescaline, psilocybin, and lysergic acid diethylamide (commonly known as LSD). These psychedelic drugs are being widely used not only by chemists and physicians, but by philosophers and theologians. Should man tamper with his mind or use drugs as the key to inner knowledge about himself? What are the moral and spiritual implications? This is indeed an important field for future research.[65]

The red-speckled mushroom *Amanita muscaria*, found in Europe, northern Asia, and in the United States, is believed by Robert Graves to have been responsible for hallucinogenic phenomena associated with Greek mystery cults related to the god Dionysus. By consuming the mushroom, participants in cult practices became capable of "fantastic bursts of muscular energy" and had the illusion of flying through the air and under the earth. The effects of the mushroom were known in Scandinavia, where amanita orgies were ritualized. A rare modern case of *A. muscaria* intoxication was reported in the Scottish Medical Journal.[66] Two brothers, salmon poachers "by trade," had for two years occasionally eaten mushrooms. Reporting on the case, Drs. McCluskie and Horne noted that this mushroom has been thought by some authorities to have been the original ambrosia or "food of the gods." "In these days of drugs, pep pills, and 'goof balls,' it was most refreshing to encounter a revival of addiction to the old ambrosia." Usually the mushrooms gave the brothers pleasant feelings of unreality and detachment. They felt an increase in power and a degree of invulnerability. On the occasion that brought them to the notice of Western Infirmary in Glasgow, they had boiled about 20 mushrooms and flavored the mixture with beer. One brother, who ate the lion's share of the concoction, was admitted to the hospital in a drowsy and confused state. After several hours, he became restless and confused and began to have auditory and visual hallucinations. He saw the skins of those round his bed peeling off in layers; his own skin began to peel. He found that by using certain words, his skin ceased to peel but that of others peeled more rapidly. He was agitated; it was impossible to communicate with him. "This stage lasted for an hour, and he then became fully conscious and reasonably well oriented. . . . His progress was good, and he was discharged on the fifth day." The brothers volunteered the information that a drink containing equal parts of amanita juice and vodka was sold in some London cafes; the drink was called a Catherine because Catherine the Great was reputed to have been an *A. muscaria* addict.

The hallucinatory effects of mescaline have been employed for centuries in the religious rites of the Southwest Indians, who chew it in its native form of peyotl cactus buttons. The crude cactus contains more than ten alkaloids: among them are bufotenine, said to be also the chief effective agent of the *A. muscaria*, and mescaline, the pure alkaloid form of which was isolated in 1894 and since been synthesized. The cactus buttons can be chewed, ground up and placed in gelatine capsules, or rolled into balls. The buttons cost from half a cent in Texas to 50 cents in New York; peyote is often referred to as "the button," "tops," a "moon," "cactus," "the bad seed," or simply as "P." Mescaline, obtainable illicitly as a crystalline powder for 50 cents to $7 per capsule, is sometimes called "Mesc" or "Big Chief."[67] Mescaline is chemically similar to amphetamine and epinephrine; its effects have been attributed to interference with the epinephrine cycle. "It is particularly noteworthy that not only LSD and mescaline but ergotropic agents in general, including amphetamine and ephedrine, when given in sufficiently large doses, induce aberrant behavior and illusions in man."[68]

Albert Hofmann, a Swiss chemist, was one of the cosynthesizers of lysergic acid diethylamide, an ergot derivative, in 1938. Five years later, while working with the same substance, he noted unusual psychic disturbances in himself.

On a Friday afternoon, April 16th, 1943, I was seized in the laboratory by a peculiar sensation of vertigo and restlessness. Objects in my vicinity and also the shape of my co-workers in the laboratory appeared to undergo optical changes. I was incapable of concentrating my mind on my work. In a dreamlike state I left the laboratory and went home where I was seized by an irresistible urge to lie down and sleep. Daylight was felt as being unpleasantly intense. I drew the curtains and immediately fell into a peculiar state of 'drunkenness,' characterized by an exaggerated imagination. With closed eyes, fantastic pictures of extraordinary plasticity and intensive kaleidoscopic colorfulness seemed to surge towards me. After two hours this state gradually subsided and I ate dinner with good appetite feeling perfectly normal and fresh.[69]

Three days later, he administered to himself 250 micrograms of LSD and found that the symptoms reappeared, this time with greater intensity. LSD is considered the most potent of the hallucinogenic drugs; the similarity between the hallucinatory and perception-distorting effects of the drug and the symptoms reported by some schizophrenics led to an early conclusion that this drug could produce a "model psychosis" and led to experimental studies, those in the United States commencing in the late 1940's.

Much of the rationale behind these experiments centered around the concept of 'model psychosis.' Through studies of the drug-induced psychotic states . . . it was hoped that an experimental analog of schizophrenia might be provided. Investigations attempted to relate the actions of LSD and mescaline to specific neurophysiologic processes and to various brain biochemical systems. . . . However, it must be acknowledged that these hopes have not been fulfilled. Currently, there is no agreement among investigators that the states produced by LSD and related drugs are phenomenologically and psychodynamically different from schizophrenia. While these drugs have provided valuable stimuli to research on the central nervous system, the mechanisms underlying their actions remain unknown.[70]

The drug as obtained through illicit channels is usually deposited on sugar cubes. It has also been distributed on animal crackers when sugar cubes treated with the drug were declared contraband, and in the Boston area it is sometimes called "crackers," although it is also called 25 (from LSD-25), "coffee" and, in Harlem "the beast," "the ghost," and "the hawk." Price ranges from $1 to $7 per sugar cube; the lower price prevails in the Boston area, which has been a center for scientific and unscientific experimentation with the drug.[71]

LSD in the early 1950's was hailed as an adjunct of psychotherapy, as hypnotism, "truth serum," and other means to circumvent patient's defenses had been. Experimentation continues, and some authorities have found the drug's use helpful, although most psychiatrists consider this a possibly harmful approach and do not utilize it in therapy. Treating 150 patients with functional psychiatric disorders, Baker in Toronto found that 100 patients were helped, although four became psychotic.[72] He found that the therapist was able to secure verbal material ordinarily difficult to elicit: the patient remembers the LSD experience and this helps his own understanding and that of the therapist in later treatment.

Levine and Ludwig have reported success in treating drug addicts with a combination of psychotherapy, LSD, and hypnosis[73]; the addicts "made dramatic claims of therapeutic benefit, expressed a strong conviction that they should remain abstinent, professed marked symptom relief, and claimed to have a new lease or outlook on life."

Gerald Klerman has discussed some of the background of the use of LSD and other "psychotomimetic" drugs to "foster personality development through 'consciousness-expansion'."[74]

Because of the unusual experiences reported by subjects under the influence of the drug, many observers speculated that these agents might provide spurs to creative thinking. Currently, the most publicized advocacy of this use of psychotomimetic drugs has come from Leary and Alpert and their associates in the International Federation for Internal Freedom (IFIF). Emphasizing mystical aspects of the drug-induced experience, they have united their psychological theories with philosophical doctrines closely allied to Zen Buddhism.

Medical and psychiatric authorities regard these drugs as psychotomimetic, i.e., producing effects similar to psychosis. . . . Furthermore, the available evidence as to possible beneficial effects in psychotherapy or personality development is limited and inconclusive. Until such evidence is forthcoming, most psychiatrists advocate that the use of these drugs should be restricted to research endeavors which incorporate careful safeguards and methodological controls.

In challenging these views, the proponents of 'consciousness-expansion' offer three arguments. First, they allege that, in their experience, these drugs have been relatively safe. Second, they state that whether psychotic-like manifestations occur depends not so much on the chemical properties of the drug but upon the attitudes of the researcher and the quality of the social environment, particularly the group setting in which the drug is given. Third, they claim that under the circumstances employed by their advocates, these drugs induce transcendent mystical experiences, thus expanding the realm of human consciousness and enhancing creativity.

Klerman counters the arguments in favor of use of these drugs to "expand consciousness" by pointing out a frequency of serious effects, such as an "experience of insanity," in 10% to 30% of experimental subjects, the lack of knowledge about dangers of chronic use, and the lack of scientific methodology in the research projects of proponents.

Alpert and Leary, controversial figures in the field of "psychedelic research" (the term *psychedelic* was introduced in 1957 by Osmond to refer to substances whose primary effect is the radical alteration of consciousness, perception, and mood), were associated with the Harvard Center for Research in Personality. Dr. Richard Alpert, a psychologist, was a member of the Harvard Social Relations Department; his associate, Dr. Timothy Leary, was a lecturer on clinical psychology.

Writing in *Look* magazine, Andrew Weil[75] has reported: that Harvard authorities were apparently unaware of the extent to which Alpert and Leary were committed to the value of the drug experience before they had done extensive testing. Both felt that the mystic insight derived from an experience with psilocybin (an active substance isolated in 1958 from the fungus known as *Psilocybe Mexicana Heim* by the same Hofmann who discovered the hallucinogenic properties of LSD) would be the solution of the emotional problems of Western man: "... only that rare Westerner we call 'mystic' or who has had a visionary experience of some sort sees clearly the game structure of behavior." After two Harvard undergraduates who had participated in the experiments required mental hospitalization, the University in 1961 secured an agreement from Alpert and Leary that no undergraduates would be used in further research. Quarrels between the two faculty members and the University administration about the continued course of their projects were reported by the undergraduate *Harvard Crimson,* one of whose staff members was unrecognized when he sat in on a private meeting for all members of the Center for Research in Personality. The deputy commissioner of the Massachusetts Health Department was drawn into the controversy, telling reporters he thought psilocybin fell into the category of drugs that had to be administered by a physician and threatening that if this turned out to be a harmful drug, those who had given it would be subject to prosecution. When Leary and Alpert openly defied the University by continuing some of their projects without meeting conditions specified by the University, the Federal Food and Drug Administration entered the matter by investigating illegal sales in Cambridge of mescaline, psilocybin, and LSD. After numerous complications, threats, charges, and countercharges, Leary disappeared from Cambridge and turned up in Los Angeles; he was promptly relieved of teaching duties and his salary stopped. "Couriers were now bringing drugs to Harvard each weekend, and more and more students were experimenting for themselves to see if Alpert and Leary had the right idea. One could arrange to buy marihuana and mescaline in local sandwich shops. The newest fad . . . was the consumption of morning-glory seeds, supposed to cause visions and all the rest." On May 27, 1963, President Nathan Pusey announced that Alpert had been fired, the first faculty firing since he had taken over the presidency ten years before.

The *Journal of the American Medical Association* reports current widespread use of bootlegged psychotomimetics. It has been repeatedly brought out that illicit use of the drugs is common in major cities on the East and West coasts, not only among college students but also among artists, writers, "beatniks," and others. A black market in LSD-25 and psilocybin exists in many metropolitan areas. There has been an unprecedented rise in the sale of seeds of a number of species of morning-glory plants. An alarming number of college students have experimented with nutmeg, stramonium and other agents that distort or alter mental functioning.[76]

The Psychedelic Review has appeared, carrying articles on "Therapeutic Use of LSD with Terminal Cancer Patients" and "The Treatment of Frigidity with LSD and Ritalin." Its publishers quote Timothy Leary and also Aldous Huxley, who felt that psychedelic drugs could provide "a gratuitous grace." Huston Smith, professor of religion and philosophy at the Massachusetts Institute of Technology, has pointed out the possibility that many of the religious perspectives of the ancients may have had a psychedelic origin, quoting such authorities as Henri Bergson and Robert Graves to this effect.[77] He describes the doctoral research project of a Harvard student; an objective description of traditional religious experiences was found to have nine characteristics. Psilocybin was administered to ten theology students and professors and a placebo to a group of ten controls at—the audacity of the experimental design commands amazement—a Good Friday service. The ten subjects who had received the psilocybin were discovered to have described their experiences in terms that met all the criteria on the traditional religious experience.

Meanwhile, Dr. Charles Dahlberg has charged that LSD has been withheld from reputable psychiatric experimenters and that only if they were working on a National Institute of Mental Health grant would they be supplied with the drug. "An NIMH grant is hard to come by, but the drug is not. A flourishing black market supplied from Europe, under-the-counter chemists, and a variety of other sources keeps in business untrained mystics, thrill seekers, and others who do not have a reputation to lose or a malpractice suit to worry about. In other words, the conscientious scientist is shackled; the quack is free to play around."[78]

New York, in 1965, added a new provision to its mental hygiene law providing for a special license to physicians for a stated period of time if they possess or dispense hallucinogenic drugs.[79] The licenses are issued only for scientific and medical reasons; the drugs covered by the law are stramonium, mescaline or peyote, lysergic acid diethylamide, and psilocybin.

Besides use of drugs to expand consciousness and increase creativity, work goes on to discover drugs to enhance learning and improve memory. Ribonucleic acid derived from yeast apparently improves memory in aged (but not senile) patients—perhaps giving some rationale for the popularity of Brewer's yeast with food faddists. Pharmaceutic researchers Glasky, Simon, and Plotnikoff have reported on the effects of magnesium pemoline, a drug that increases the activity of the enzyme involved in the production of ribonucleic acid in the brain cells and leads to increased memory and learning power in experimental animals.[80]

Just as scientific advances in eugenics, population control, human experimentation, organ grafting, and other aspects of modern medicine raise questions that cut across disciplinary lines and involve lawyer, legislator, research scientist, medical clinician, theologian, and philosopher, so too the use of drugs to control or augment the mind represents an area where planning, based on the present determination of what kind of society we wish to achieve and how to progress towards it, is needed. Here scientific advances and new scientific knowledge outdistance society's ability suitably to use and control the new agents and methods. We read of the communications crisis and the population crisis, the technologic growth crisis and the distribution crisis, the control of instruments of warfare crisis and the moral crisis. Behind all the other crises is the values crisis—the need for society to determine what values it feels are important in an increasingly complex world and the need for these values to be translated into acceptable codes and workable laws.

CHAPTER 17

Doctor and Patient: Whose Doctor?

How happy is he born and taught,
That serveth not another's will;
Whose armour is his honest thought
And simple truth his utmost skill!

SIR HENRY WOTTON, contemporary of Shakespeare, was not advising doctors when he wrote "The Character of a Happy Life." Instead, he was praising the independent unwordly life spent in moral pursuits. But the philosophy of independence, of being one's own master and of indignantly refusing to serve "another's will," has long been a part of medical tradition.

Studies of the personalities of medical students indicate that one of the chief motives that influences them in their choice of profession is the opportunity that medicine offers to be "self-employed," to be free of the necessity of working in the more authoritarian world of corporation or civil service, or in social work or teaching, where one works under supervisors and superiors.

Tending to be conservative politically, physicians have viewed with alarm any proposals that would change them from independent entrepreneurs to interdependent parts of complex social schemes. On the grounds that their traditional independence would be lost, they have opposed governmental insurance plans for the medical or hospital care of the aged and the increasing influence of research-oriented hospitals connected to medical schools, where staff physicians, who both treat and teach, receive salaries. "Fee for service," payment for each task performed for a patient rather than by salary, has been the watchword of the independent-minded doctor. Plans to put a hospital's doctors on salary, even when the doctor is a pathologist or radiologist and so not directly involved in a relationship with patients, have led to threats of hospital boycotts, legal actions and other vigorous actions, by doctors who see any proposal to substitute a salaried for a piece-work basis as an attack on the traditional relationship of doctor to patient as well as a step towards further inroads on their independence.

Doctors who fight against a salaried status claim that the payer of the salary—hospital, agency, or branch of the government—can influence medical decisions concerning the patient and thus alter the doctor-patient relationship. When health insurance plans were first proposed, even those as apparently innocuous as Blue Cross, they were opposed for the same reason. The opposition to private insurance has dissipated, but doctors continue to oppose government insurance plans, such as Medicare; they voice the fear that the insurer can exert pressure on the doctor who accepts insurance money.

While doctors fight vigorously for "fee for service" and the elimination of third-party relationships on some fronts, on others they have given over the fight long since, and no opposition voices are heard. For more than a hundred years, the psychiatrists who treat the bulk of hospitalized psychiatric patients in state and other hospitals have been on salary. Municipal hospitals treating the indigent have salaried doctors, and there is little protest against the use of salaried physicians in the military, Veterans Administration, Public Health Service, prisons and other institutions, and by industrial corporations and business.

The intervention of such third parties as private insurance companies, which have come to pay a third of all doctors' fees,[1] is now encouraged. The protest heard now is primarily against the extension of third-party medicine in private and teaching hospitals and the extension of government insurance plans. Yet the *New England Journal of Medicine* points out that "clergymen, college professors, ship captains and judges, on a professional plane not greatly below that to which the physician aspires, appear untroubled by their failure to be compensated on a fee-for-service basis." It notes that organized medicine has "fought with stubborn vigor—and generally unsuccessfully—against the interposition of third parties in the paying of compensation, whether by voluntary prepayment health insurance plans or by salary. This resistance has been directed even against plans that included payment of fee for service, if a third party was involved. The gradual giving ground by the profession, under protest, has so far resulted in new and not necessarily unacceptable methods of delivering medical care, with no apparent sacrifice on the part of either physician or patient."[2]

Psychiatry is involved in fee for service and the role of third parties in ways that differ from the involvement of the rest of medicine. Paradoxically, the psychiatrist, in a capacity such as employee of a state hospital, has anticipated the trend towards salary rather than fee, while as a private practitioner, he has felt strongly that unless the patient pays a fee, preferably from his own funds and that represents some sacrifice on his part, he will undervalue the importance of the treatment. In regard to their relationship to insurance companies which pay part of the patient's bill, psychiatrists have also been in a position different from other doctors', first, because insurance companies pay nothing or only a small percentage of the costs of most psychiatric treatment, and second, because the confidentiality involved in the doctor-patient relationship makes cooperation with insurance companies difficult when drug or alcohol addiction, sexual deviation, psychosis, and similar disorders—rather than gallstones or a hernia—are the conditions under treatment.

Let us go a little more deeply into the subject of how the involvement of third parties—insurers, employers of the physician, employers of the patient, and others—affects the relationship of doctor and patient in medicine generally and in psychiatry particularly. We can start, as we often start in medical discussions, with Hippocrates (or, rather, the code of medical ethics which bears his name).

Although the Hippocratic Oath was once administered as a formal oath, it is not formally sworn to by most contemporary physicians. Now it is usually honored as an expression of an ethical code that a doctor implicitly accepts in assuming his professional role. In the event of a doctor's delinquency, it asks a terrible retribution: ". . . as I am faithful to this my oath, may happiness and good repute be ever mine—the opposite if I shall be forsworn."

The oath is simplicity itself on the score of the relationship of doctor and patient; the doctor vows "that I will exercise my art solely for the cure of my patients. . . ."

What was obviously contemplated in the days of Hippocrates was a one-to-one relationship where the doctor owed a duty only to the patient. Probably kings and emperors were the earliest of the "third parties," who hired a doctor to examine but not necessarily to treat; the government has in modern times become the largest employer of physicians for purposes of both classification, such as draft examinations, and treatment. Third-party relationships, which involved doctor, patient, plus an employer who pays the doctor and deserves some consideration from him, fall into two main categories: the doctor treats the patient in a way approximating the normal one-to-one doctor-patient relationship, but a third party pays all or part of the doctor's fee or salary; or, the doctor is a nontreating physician whose function is administrative: to diagnose, classify and advise—particularly on whether to hire or fire—rather than to treat.

When a patient is being treated by a doctor, he usually feels that a legal relationship has arisen, involving undertaking of treatment by the doctor, consent to the treatment by the patient, the right to have confidences preserved, and the right to have the doctor act solely in the patient's interest. The presence of a third party alters the relationship; the doctor now has a duty to the patient *and* to the third party. Doctors know many "pseudo third parties"—parties who have no legal right to be involved but because they can exert pressure still have to be consulted. Family, friends, and those with power to affect the patient financially, such as his employer, are not third parties unless they pay the patient's bills, but they still sometimes demand information, advise the doctor, and act like real third parties. Insurance companies liable for the patient's medical bills and—in the case of corporation or government doctors—those responsible for the doctor's salary are more directly interested third parties.

Insurance companies may be involved in any of three ways. Rarely, they may be involved because they insure the doctor and thus alter his plan of treatment for the patient. More commonly, they are involved as the patient's insurer, which requires confidential material about the patient and sometimes sets up concerning reimbursement regulations that affect the treatment plan. They may also be involved as a "pseudo third party"—not a third party in the legal sense, but nevertheless an intruder—either because a damage suit is pending and they want information to defend it, or because the patient wants to take out life insurance and they want to know if the condition for which he is being treated increases their risk.

The employer of a salaried doctor may be involved. The doctor who does draft board examinations, the alienist who reports to the court on the ability of a prisoner to stand trial or tell right from wrong, military service physicians, industrial physicians employed by companies to treat employees, salaried staff of medical or psychiatric hospitals, prison doctors, whether they treat patients or advise parole and pardon boards—all have a split allegiance. These doctors may treat the patient, merely examine him and report to a third party, or combine functions of treating and nontreating physician.

The patient's boss is a "pseudo third party" who makes his presence felt. He often requires information on his condition and its prognosis before allowing the patient to return to work. Schools similarly seek information regarding students. The patient signs a release authorizing the doctor to furnish information, but he usually is not aware whether or not the information the doctor furnishes will be damaging. The doctor cannot refuse to furnish the information without prejudicing the patient in the eyes of this "third party." Besides the obvious issue of confidentiality, other pressures may be exerted. An employee may be allowed to return to his job only if he promises to continue in psychiatric treatment.

The issues of privacy, of the right to have the doctor act solely in the interest of the patient, and of the other concomitants of the traditional doctor-patient relationship, also involve other disciplines—psychology and penology, for instance—that become allied with medicine in the treatment or classification of the patient. A doctor asks a patient to take a psychological test; a governmental agency asks an employee to take a lie-detector test; police authority requires a determination of alcohol or barbiturate level in the blood. The physician may be treating or merely advising a third party on an administrative determination. Does the special nature of the doctor-patient relationship encompass the patient's relationships with other personnel, when the results of such encounters may finally become part of a medical evaluation?

Let us commence with some of the problems involving insurance. A rare medical/legal situation, which perhaps illustrates the extent to which some physicians can be influenced by third parties in their dealing with patients, was recently heard in Ohio.[3] The plaintiff was a hospital patient whose bed had collapsed; he sued the hospital for his resulting damages. The insurance company that insured the hospital was the insurer also for the patient's personal physician. According to the allegations of the patient, the insurance company falsely told the doctor that a suit was planned against him, as well as the hospital, and on the basis of this threat the doctor turned over to the insurance company the patient's complete file and terminated treatment of the patient. The patient-plaintiff alleged that he was deprived of the treatment of the physician best qualified to help him, and that he had also had his suit against the hospital prejudiced by the disclosure of the confidential information.

The court criticized the physician on both scores, saying that when a patient selects a physician to treat him "he does so with the full expectation that such physician will do his best to restore him to health, and the contract into which they enter is deserving of more attention than a businessman's expectation of profit from a purely commercial transaction. The physician-patient contract is not purely commercial and should not permit a third party to effect its rupture."

Less flagrant but more usual effects of pressure on the part of insurance companies arise from rules and regulations regarding reimbursement of fees to doctors. Sometimes the insurance company rules determine the frequency and duration of psychiatric treatment. The insurance payments often make treatment possible when the patient would not be able to afford private therapy, but, in exchange, the doctor gives up some of his freedom to plan treatment and to guard confidences. An insurance policy may specify that the patient will be reimbursed for 50% of psychiatric charges, but that the maximum reimbursement is $5 weekly. The psychiatrist would like to see the patient every second week for a one-hour appointment and bill him at the usual rate of $20. Only a fourth of the patient's bill will be covered by insurance, then, but if the psychiatrist alters his plan and sees the patient weekly for half-hour visits at $10, in spite of the fact that he sees the patient for the same amount of time during the course of a month and the patient's bills are the same in each instance, the insurance now covers half the treatment. Sometimes the determination to treat a patient as an outpatient or a hospitalized inpatient is governed by the terms of the insurance he carries.

Besides determining, to some extent, the type of treatment, frequency and duration, third parties have the ability to secure confidential information from doctors. As a condition prerequisite to reimbursement, an insurance company will want information from the doctor about the patient. The patient may not want confidential information passed on to the insurance company, but he has no alternative if he wants to be reimbursed; the doctor may have as a principle the maintenance of strict confidentiality, but if he fails to submit information, his patient is not reimbursed.

Most psychiatrists do not feel obligated to be strictly truthful in reporting medical information to insurance companies, or to such a "pseudo third party" as the employer of the patient, who has no legal relationship with the doctor. An insurance company is often told that a patient has a neurotic depression despite the psychiatrist's feeling that the depression is really of psychotic proportions; the physician does not have control over the ultimate use of the information he supplies, and he prefers to keep potentially damaging information out of the office files of third parties, whose office personnel may not feel bound by his code concerning confidentiality. An alcoholic employee, who has missed time at work, is told that he cannot return to his job until he sees a psychiatrist, and gets a statement from the psychiatrist saying that he is able to work consistently. The psychiatrist has three choices —of nobly refusing to supply information, which will mean that the patient continues on an unpaid vacation; of honestly saying that the patient will very possibly continue to get into trouble if he returns to the job, since he has not mastered the problem, which will also mean that the patient continues on vacation; or of optimistically saying that probably the patient can once again function in the work situation. The horns of the psychiatrist's dilemma are the choices between honestly injuring the patient or of dishonestly protecting him.

Henry Davidson has frankly described how state mental hospitals, in their staff conferences where the diagnoses of patients are discussed, are influenced by such considerations as the patient's employment. A schoolteacher, for instance, will not get her job back on recovery if the ominous diagnosis of schizophrenia has been used; so a milder diagnosis is substituted.[4]

Life insurance companies provide a particularly difficult problem for the psychiatrist. A patient, or a former patient, has applied for life insurance and has passed his physical examination; in zealous accuracy, he has listed the name of his psychiatrist among the doctors whom he has consulted within the last five years. The insurance company, armed with a permission for release of information from the patient, sends a request for information, (together with a check for $2 or $3 to "reimburse" the doctor for his "inconvenience" or a statement that the physician should submit a bill if the token fee is unsatisfactory). The psychiatrist knows that if he states that the patient was treated for a serious psychiatric condition, the insurance may not be issued; moreover, the patient will be able to pinpoint the psychiatrist's report as the bar to his receiving a policy, since he has already passed the insurance physical examination. Under the circumstances, the psychiatrist may describe the condition as minor, and cash the $2 check.

When an insurance company wants information about a doctor's patient or former patient, not because it will reimburse the patient for fees but because of a business matter—an application for a policy or perhaps a pending law-suit—doctors may feel strongly about not providing information, but since the patient has signed a permission for release of information, and since the doctor does not want to prejudice the insurance company against his patient, he usually supplies the information under unspoken protest.

An internist has described the effect of another third-party arrangement—a government agency's or a corporation's employing a physician to treat other employees—on the sort of medicine practiced:

A few weeks after I started practice, when I had more time than money or patients, I was offered a part-time job in the dispensary of a railroad company that operates its own closed-panel health plan. When I reported for work, I saw a long line of patients waiting.

The nurse told me, "We have to see these patients fast—40 or 50 an hour." She pointed to shelves of prepared medications, each with a label like "Headache Pills," "Cough Syrup," "Stomach Pills." "We just give them one of these medicines," she said, "depending on what they complain about."

I quit the job immediately. . . .[5]

Sometimes the salaried physician who sees a patient does not regard himself as the patient's doctor, but merely as a classifier and an agent in an administrative process. The draft board doctor, for example, asks the prospective draftee whether he likes girls not to help him in his psychosexual development, but to enable the doctor's employer—the draft board—to choose those to select and those to reject for the armed services. Or, an Army doctor is asked to interview a soldier who has refused to perform assigned duties or who has been arrested for a punishable offense; the soldier will be tried, but before the trial begins a medical or psychiatric report is ordered. As a result of the doctor's examination, the soldier will be offered a discharge for the convenience of the government, ordered to stand trial, or be sent to a hospital. Neither the soldier, who is the patient, nor the doctor-officer can tell at the start of the examination whether the doctor is acting as part of an administrative process or is initiating a treatment process, and neither can tell whether the patient is wise or foolish in being nondefensive and revealing himself completely to the doctor.

Courts have held that when one merely submits to a physical examination (as one prerequisite to employment or to securing insurance) by a doctor employed by another, there is no real doctor-patient relationship. The doctor is not under any duty, for example, to discover a disease that the patient may have. The patient may have tuberculosis, but the doctor who does the physical examination cannot be sued later, when this becomes apparent, because he did not do a sufficiently thorough examination. This limitation of duty to the patient is said to result from the physician's employment contract and lack of relationship to the examinee: the physician's primary duty is to his employer. If, however, the doctor does discover a physical disorder in an employment or preemployment examination, he probably does have the duty to disclose his finding to the examinee, and if the patient suffers damages as a result of not having been told of his condition, the doctor's employer would probably be liable. In the case of an insurance examination, the law is similar; the main difference is that even if a medical problem is discovered, the doctor will not reveal its nature to the patient, but, instead, will advise him to be examined by his personal physician. He may go so far as to tell the patient to have the personal physician get in touch with the company medical director or himself.[6] A monograph of the Law Department of the American Medical Association gives the business philosophy that underlies this practice.

One might wonder why an insurer would not permit an examining physician to disclose to the applicant his findings. The answer is that the insurer and applicant are carrying on negotiations concerning the insurance contract, and the physician, as the agent of the insurer, has no right to interfere in any way with the negotiations. For example, he might tell X that X is certainly a class A risk, but the insurer's medical director may come to a different conclusion. X then expects to be paying premiums as a class A risk but is offered a policy demanding class C premiums and refuses it. On the other hand, the examiner might tell X that with his health he could never obtain insurance, causing X to cancel his application.[7]

In the case of the insurance examination or the preemployment or predraft physical examination, the patient (who more properly can be called the examinee, because he has not acquired patient status) usually realizes that a doctor-patient relationship does not exist, although if a doctor starts to ask probing questions about psychiatric problems, he may find that the authority of the doctor's position is sufficient to induce him to disclose information that ordinarily is disclosed only when there is a doctor-patient relationship. But many situations arise with nontreating physicians and employee physicians that seem to give rise to some kind of doctor-patient relationship, even though the patient may not have hired the doctor, may have no confidence in him, may feel that he will not work in the patient's own interest, and may have no financial responsibility for paying for his services.

Here are some additional situations involving third-party employers of examining doctors never foreseen by Hippocrates.

A trainee in the Labor Department's Youth Opportunity Program, who is apparently doing satisfactory work, takes a routine personality inventory test, and, on the basis of the results, is asked to see the Program's consulting psychiatrist.[8]

An orderly working in a hospital operating room is felt by some of the personnel to be erratic in his work and overly familiar towards nurses, and is required to visit the hospital's outpatient psychiatric clinic.

A prison psychiatrist is told by a prisoner that he has committed a crime that the police still list as unsolved.

A company physician treats an employee who admits that he is an alcoholic.

An Army doctor deals with a patient who has fears that he will go berserk.

A prison doctor sees an anxious patient but is prevented by prison rules from prescribing tranquilizers.

A psychiatrist examines an admitted murderer to see whether he is competent to stand trial.

In all these cases, in varying degrees, the doctor's allegiance is divided—he owes a duty to someone other than the patient. The physician, especially the psychiatrist, is in the anomalous position of asking the patient to be completely frank and open, to give details of venereal illnesses, sexual promiscuity, undiscovered legal offenses, in the interest of the doctor-patient relationship, at the same time that *he* owes a duty to an employer to use some of this information in a manner adverse to the best interest of the patient. Perhaps a psychiatrist interviewing a prospective employee for the Peace Corps or the Youth Opportunity Program should have a sign prominently displayed: "Ordinary Rules Governing Relationship of Doctor and Patient Do Not Apply: Anything You Say May Be Used Against You."

The sign should read, at least: "Proceed With Caution." Surely it should not have to read: "Abandon Hope, All Ye Who Enter Here."

In the case of the prison psychiatrist who is told by a prisoner of a crime still unsolved, Dr. Henry Davidson feels that most psychiatrists would value the doctor-patient relationship more than their duty to the prison, and would reveal information disclosed during therapy only in the case of unsolved attacks against prison guards and personnel and when a jail break or other major disturbance is being planned.[9] Even drawing the line this far towards the side of confidentiality in the doctor-patient relationship leaves some unanswered questions. Although the doctor knows that he will not harm his patient by disclosure, can the patient accept the reassurances of the doctor and speak in the uncensored way that psychiatrists desire? What happens when the psychiatrist who has developed a good therapeutic alliance with a prisoner (a difficult and not altogether common circumstance) is told by the prisoner about antisocial attitudes, and the same psychiatrist—having taken off his therapist cap and donned the cap of parole board consultant—is asked to recommend the prisoner for release?

The most notorious instance of a nontreating physician with allegiances to others beside the patient involved a military hero as the patient, a psychiatrist who not only did not treat but never went to see his patient as the doctor, and the brother of the President of the United States as a third party. More than 2,500 complaints, two of them from county medical societies, were received by the American Medical Association against the physician, Dr. Charles E. Smith, Medical Director and Chief Psychiatrist of the Federal Bureau of Prisons.[10] Many of the complaints were members of the "radical right" spurred into action by the fact that the nontreated patient was former Major General Edwin Walker. Liberals and others interested in civil rights and liberties despite the General's involvement in this matter by allegedly leading a demonstration against civil rights for Negroes—were also among the protestants.[11]

General Walker had fought against integration of the University of Mississippi (Ole' Miss) and had been arrested for his pains. Dr. Smith was asked by the Department of Justice if, on the basis of what he knew about the case from newspaper and television accounts, he thought he could reasonably make a statement about the General's mental condition. He was given an Associated Press report of the University of Mississippi incident, a transcript of six-month-old testimony by the General on military preparedness before a Senate subcommittee, news clippings of previous activities of the General, and some of the General's army medical records covering the period 1927 to 1958. On the basis of this information, which he reviewed that night in the office of Robert Kennedy, the Attorney General, the doctor signed an affidavit concerning the General's state of mental health:

Some of his reported behavior reflects sensitivity and essentially unpredictable and seemingly bizarre outbursts of the type often observed in individuals suffering with paranoid mental disorder. There are also indications in his medical history of functional and psychosomatic disorders which could be precursors of the more serious disorder which his present behavior suggests. From this and other information available to me I believe his recent behavior has been out of keeping with that of a person of his station, background, and training, and that as such it may be indicative of an underlying mental disturbance.

The affidavit, besides being an example of the political use of medical opinion, is a commentary on the confidentiality of Army records.

On the same day that the memorandum was prepared and put in affidavit form, it was used to support a motion, filed by the government in the United States District Court for the Northern District of Mississippi, to have General Walker committed to a psychiatric hospital for a mental examination. Meantime, the General had been transferred to the Springfield Medical Center for federal prisoners in Missouri, and the court directed that a psychiatric examination be done at that institution; it did not fix a time limit for the confinement of the patient-prisoner but stated only that he should be held in Springfield until the examination was completed. The examination of a psychiatrist filed two weeks later resulted in a report that the General was neither insane nor incompetent.

In response to the 2,500 complaints to the AMA, its Judicial Council opened an investigation into the matter and in its course consulted three psychiatrists (whose names were not released) as well as the AMA Council of Mental Health and the American Psychiatric Association. All of these agreed that the doctor had not violated any of the formal Principles of Medical Ethics, despite the doctor's rendering his medical opinion in Washington, DC, while the patient was in Mississippi and Missouri. It was also agreed that the affidavit that Dr. Smith had given was not a medical diagnosis, although what it was was never clarified. The only light on this in the Judicial Council Opinion is: "Some expressed the opinion that he had given an impression or opinion based on information given to him. In this connection, it was pointed out that physicians are frequently called upon by attorneys or courts to render a professional opinion to assist the court in deciding a technical point. It is then the court's responsibility to evaluate such opinion." The Council concluded that Doctor Smith "did not violate professional confidence and did not make a diagnosis in regard to the mental condition of General Walker."

The Judicial Council added this addendum:

The Judicial Council expresses concern about possible future situations wherein a physician might be subject to political control in order to pervert his medical opinion or be used as a tool for political purposes. The Council urges physicians to be alert to such possibilities and to refuse to give such opinions which might be used for political purposes.

That the suggestion in Dr. Smith's affidavit—that the General was displaying symptoms seen in individuals with "paranoid mental disorder" and probably suffering from this condition—was not diagnostic does not seem credible. To befog the issue by saying it was merely informational and a nondiagnostic opinion would imply criticism of the court, which was not empowered to hear a motion for judicial determination of mental competency unless the United States Attorney could show reasonable cause for belief that the prisoner was either insane or so incompetent as to be unable to understand the legal proceedings in which he was involved.

More recently, 2,417 psychiatrists responded to a magazine poll concerning Senator Goldwater's mental stability during a presidential campaign; the majority stated that they saw indications of personality disturbance and instability. Organized medical groups, taking a position diametrically opposed to the Judicial Council in General Walker's case, stated that such opinions or diagnoses should be condemned. Dr. Donovan Ward, then president of the AMA, in an official statement for that organization said, that "a physician can properly arrive at a medical opinion on the health of an individual only by following accepted clinical procedures, including personal examination of the patient."[12]

The greatest complexity in psychiatric opinion is not long-range diagnoses nor pressure to use medical opinion for political ends. Instead, it is the fact that starting on a medical basis—the examination by alienists of criminals who appeared to be mentally unbalanced, and the work of Freud and his followers with technics involving depth exploration of the psyche, using free association and uncensored stream of consciousness—the application of dynamic psychology has spread out to include psychological testing, use of psychiatric interview technics by psychologists and social workers, and psychiatric treatment by nonmedical personnel (usually, once again, psychologists and social workers).

How much of the protection to the doctor-patient relationship that results from ethics, tradition and law carries over into allied fields? How much of the raw data elicited by nonphysicians but utilized in a process employing physicians as final arbiters or review authorities is encompassed within the topic of relationship of patient to doctor? The complexity of the relationships between medicine and nonmedical fields is evidenced by the history of the development of psychological testing by both medical and nonmedical people, which tests are used to elicit material that may be used by medical, paramedical or nonmedical personnel and that may or may not be part of a treatment or classification process where psychiatrists may participate fully, or as advisors, or not at all. The tests most used today were developed by physicians, who used them as part of treatment (example, Herman Rorschach), and psychologists, who used them for classification and research into learning theory (example, David Wechsler). Once developed, the tests came to be used extensively by psychiatrists, psychologists or others for diagnosis, information concerning psychodynamics, possible indications as to prognosis, and for help in treatment; they have come to be used extensively by similar categories of people for entirely non-therapeutic purposes, such as vocational guidance, hiring and firing, school placement.

A psychologist, for better or worse, is not the equivalent of a psychiatrist; much of his work may be theoretic and research-oriented, and he does testing and undertakes other functions for which he has had special training. Psychiatrists do work not open to psychologists; they may prescribe medicine and give electric shock treatment, and their training has been with patients to an extent not realizable in the training of other disciplines. Nevertheless, in a wide area the work of the clinical psychologist and the psychiatric therapist overlap, and there is no major distinction between the two disciplines. When psychiatrists are unavailable for difficult or underpaid jobs, such as therapy in homes for delinquents or the mentally retarded or in prisons, psychologists are hired to do the work. The psychologist will not dispense drugs, and he is working theoretically under medical supervision; but since many psychiatrists try to be sparing in prescribing drugs and the supervision is often largely fictitious, the work consists of therapy, writing progress and prognostic reports, and making disposition recommendations largely on his own. The patient often has not made the distinction between the two professions, and may refer to his doctor as belonging to one profession when in reality he belongs to the other. (Even judges are often unable to make the distinction.) Whether the patient is seeing a psychologist or a psychiatrist, he may decide to trust "the doctor" implicitly and to produce uncensored material as Freud proposed. He may even "free associate"—follow the basic Freudian rule of saying whatever comes to mind if his therapist favors this analytic technic—and in the process produce material that he would not produce if he did not feel that the relationship was a doctor-patient relationship and protected.

The merging of psychiatric and psychological testimony for legal purposes has been advanced, with, once again, Judge Bazelon writing the majority decision. In *Jenkins* vs *United States*,[13] the United States Court of Appeals for the District of Columbia has ruled that even though they lack medical training, experienced clinical psychologists are qualified to render expert testimony as to mental disorder; one of the criteria for accepting their testimony—illustrating the union of psychologist and psychiatrist in the diagnostic process—was that the psychologists whose testimony had been the subject of dispute in this case "regularly reported their diagnostic conclusions to psychiatrists ultimately responsible for treatment of the patient."

The question, then, concerns the merging in modern life of testing methods and therapeutic efforts by psychiatry and psychology. Are psychologists who act like psychiatrists bound by the medical, ethical and legal standards that govern the doctor-patient relationship? Is a physician who uses psychological test results and who asks his patient —soldier, prisoner, job applicant, employee, private patient—to take tests entitled to use the results to the detriment of the patient?

Writing in *The New Republic*, James Ridgeway says that applicants for government jobs and employees of government agencies are "run through batteries of psychological tests meant to reveal some latent sex deviation. The personnel people, who apparently have come to imagine they are psychiatrists, bother employees with silly, indecent questions about the workings of their private parts. . . ."[14]

Although "the personnel people" are probably not psychiatrists and possibly not psychologists, they are drawing on the body of psychiatric-psychological knowledge in order to test and to formulate hypotheses about the psychic lives, with emphasis on sexual deviation and loyalty, of the job applicants. This may often be unfortunate and sometimes be unwise, but it is ubiquitous and derived from the model of the doctor-patient relationship. In other situations—such as interpretation of test results, evaluating reports, mass screening, interviewing dubious prospects, applying and interpreting physiologic testing devices—such as the polygraph lie-detector, which is expected to use body changes to trap devious job applicants—there are situations where doctors actively enter into the process of interviewing, hiring and firing. Writes Ridgeway:

Sometimes, however, the hunters of homosexuals get caught up in their own machinery. Lie detectors, gadgets which register emotional reactions and are used by various agencies to screen out undesirables, now are suspected of actually turning away conscientious virile Americans so badly needed by the CIA for spying. (It turns out that normal young men may be nervous about revealing details of their sex life and end up flunking these tests, while homosexuals, who are less fearful about theirs, pass with flying colors.)

One woman employee applying for the Foreign Service was told to answer, "quickly and without thinking or deliberation," the following, true or false:
Once in a while I think of things too bad to talk about.
My sex life is satisfactory.
Evil spirits possess me at times.
I have never been in trouble because of my sex behavior.
I am very strongly attracted by members of my own sex.
I believe in a life hereafter.
I have never indulged in any unusual sex practices.
I read the Bible several times a week.
There is something wrong with my sex organs.

Psychological tests used in personnel determination may seem far afield from the doctor-patient relationship. Yet these tests were devised by doctors and psychologists for use in working with patients, they are administered by nondoctors under the supervision and with the consultative efforts of doctors, and the potential employee who answers such questions in an atypical way is then interviewed by doctors who have access to this information.

Time Magazine has printed a more complete list of the questions of the Minnesota Multiphasic Personality Inventory.[15]

At the Departments of State, Labor, and Health Education & Welfare, the Export-Import Bank, the Peace Corps, and, of all things, the Bonneville Power Administration, job applicants are tested for their personality as a prerequisite of employment. The tests differ, but the most widely used and the one upon which the others are based is the Minnesota Multiphasic Personality Inventory (MMPI), a 566-question, true-false quiz developed at the University of Minnesota. The test has recently come under strong congressional criticism on the ground that it requires answers that are nobody else's business.

Sample questions:
I have had very peculiar and strange experiences.
I have never been in trouble because of my sex behavior.
My soul sometimes leaves my body.
I have not lived the right kind of life.
Sometimes I am strongly attracted by the personal articles of others, such as shoes, gloves, etc. so that I want to handle or steal them though I have no use for them.
At times I have a strong urge to do something harmful or shocking.
I believe women ought to have as much sexual freedom as men.
I believe I am being followed.
I have never indulged in any unusual sex practices.
Sometimes I feel as if I must injure myself or someone else.
The top of my head sometimes feels tender.
I am worried about sex matters.
I believe my sins are unpardonable.
I brood a great deal.
I like repairing a door latch.

The *Time* article is aptly titled: "Yes, I Believe I am Being Followed."

The testing process and its connection with the profession of psychiatry, and the relationship of psychiatry to psychology, are receiving new attention. Two Senate subcommittees have probed the use of questionnaires to delve into beliefs and habits of government employees and prospective employees and of electronic devices to check employee activities; the subcommittee on constitutional rights has denounced the use of the questionnaires and noted concern over the spread of such testing to nonsensitive agencies.[16] Use of the polygraph test—the "lie detector"—by employers has drawn the fire of unions; in particular they object to pledges demanded of workers that give management the right to fire them if they refuse at any time to take a polygraph test.[17] The House Committee on Government Operations has stated that the polygraph cannot differentiate truth and falsehood.[18] The Civil Service Commission, which regulates personnel practices for nine out of ten people hired by the federal government, has recently banned personality inventory-type psychological tests.[19] Dr. Forrest L. Vance, speaking before the American Psychological Association, has called personality tests an invasion of privacy and pointed out they were developed for clinical use on a voluntary basis.[20] Henry Chauncey, president of the Educational Testing Service, has joined the list of those questioning the usefulness of the traditional IQ test as an indicator of intellectual potentiality.[21] Louis D. Cohen has stated that "experiments with the Rorschach, TAT, Draw-a-Person, Bender Gestalt, and other such instruments, continually report failure in the systematic and stable prediction of personality and/or behavior."[22] Dr. Brewster Smith, of the University of California, has reported that Peace Corps volunteers performed jobs in Ghana with a success that confounded the predictions of the psychiatrists who had rated the volunteers before they left the United States; the psychiatrists were overconcerned with adjustment and mental health and insufficiently concerned with "guts" and "ability to respond to a challenge."[23]

In the field of criminal responsibility, the kind of examination usually done by the psychiatrist has also come under fire. Thomas Flannery, Assistant United States Attorney for the District of Columbia, has told a legal seminar that psychiatrists who testify as to a defendant's sanity after only a brief interview and without knowing all the facts of the crime itself are presenting virtually worthless evidence.[24]

The invasion of privacy is an issue here, but it is not the major issue for forensic medicine or forensic psychiatry. Nor are civil liberties, as important as they are, the chief trouble maker. The crux is the dual roles and the dual allegiance of the doctor (or of the psychologist who acts like a doctor) and the inability of the patient to be sure that his doctor is acting in his best interest. The physician wears two hats, and the patient is not told which hat belongs to the physician acting as an agent of a third party and which hat belongs to the physician following the Hippocratic injunction to exercise his art solely for the cure of his patients.

The Senior Consultant to the Peace Corps and the Chief Psychiatrist, Medical Division, Peace Corps have described the complexities of that organization's psychiatric branch when, during the evaluation of an applicant who has brashly admitted that he has previously seen a psychiatrist, it proceeds to seek information from the former therapist.[25] The Peace Corps psychiatrist now not only asks the job applicant to consider him a doctor while he acts as an evaluator for his agency but also exerts pressure on doctors who have had previous contact with the job applicant to reveal the details of the therapeutic relationship. The authors note without comment that between 0.5 and 1.0% of the more than 100,000 Americans who have applied for Peace Corps service have previously seen a psychiatrist for consultation or assistance; they do not note that this figure—low in comparison with percentages of undergraduates seen by college psychiatrists at many universities—indicates that most Peace Corps applicants presumably withhold this information. They note that the request for information has presented a dilemma for psychiatrists who question the usefulness of such information as well as the appropriateness of furnishing it. Part of their answer is that "the psychotherapeutic relationship, as a model of an individual's interpersonal relationships, can provide a measure of his capacity to become effectively involved with other people and in the kinds of activities that take place in the Peace Corps, which is essentially a people-to-people activity." They see no real problem of confidentiality in requesting this information:

The Peace Corps Psychiatric Branch, in seeking information about an applicant's emotional stability, has no intention of interfering with effective psychotherapy or in learning confidential information which is unrelated to the issue at hand. It may be an extreme position, however, to operate on the assumption that a psychiatrist cannot release information about the treatment and still be true to himself or to his patient, when the patient authorizes the therapist to release the information and when the patient has consciously applied for a situation which is known to be emotionally demanding.

The authors do have the grace to admit that there may be a legitimate question just how "voluntary" the applicant's authorization for release of information may be, since if he does not sign this release "inevitably, the reviewing staff may wonder why an applicant would hesitate to permit the release of information and what he is afraid of revealing."

In a discussion of this point of view, Dr. Robert L. Arnstein, of the Yale University Student Health Service, suspects that the applicant feels he has little real choice when asked to sign the waiver. Many applicants are not worried because they feel that they have nothing to hide; "others may not be so sure that they have nothing to hide, but faced with the alternative of signing or withdrawing their Peace Corps application, I imagine that most sign the waiver in a burst of fatalism and simply hope that there will be no adverse consequences." He has other objections to the release of information.[26]

I have heard enough comment on campus to feel that if information were routinely released in such situations there would be real reluctance on the part of some (if not many) to consult our service initially or to be candid in therapy. Whether or not this is a reasonable concern on the part of the student is perhaps less important than the fact that the attitude exists. In the interests of preventive psychiatry . . . our general aim as a college health service is to make early consultation as easy as possible for the student. If we agree to a policy of releasing information, it seems to me that it is only right that the student should be so informed when he first comes in, and I feel that for some this would act as a real bar to undertaking treatment. . . .

When one has dealt with some of the ramifications of these problems, one begins to wonder whether honesty is really the best policy. One of the questions most frequently asked by student patients is, "Should I say I have seen a psychiatrist on the application?" Although I cannot really conceive of recommending dishonesty, there are moments when I am tempted, and this, I think, is an extremely unfortunate state of affairs.

One solution would be for doctors to remain free of involvement in matters of hiring and firing; another might be the clear differentiation —perhaps by using the old-fashioned term of alienist and warning the patient that the doctor was not his doctor—of the doctor who owes and does not owe a duty to the patient. Dr. Joseph Hartog has suggested that, "ideally," psychiatrists and psychologists should refuse to participate in any diagnostic procedure involving a person who is sent because of disciplinary, management or performance difficulties; but he does not find this position practical.[27]

The confusion arises when a person's emotional state or personality is said to be related to the personnel problem. In one sense, all personnel problems are psychological in origin. But so also are all crime, marital, and school problems. Yet shifting administrative or disciplinary responsibility (or in courts, judicial responsibility) onto the back of psychiatrists or psychologists directly or indirectly (by overweighing their opinions) is an unwelcome and dangerous position for the profession. This is an evident evil when a person loses his job allegedly on the basis of a psychiatric or psychological evaluation.

Dr. Hartog has his own list of questions concerning the position of the third-party psychiatrist.

Should he be the psychological rubber-stamp of his employer? Should he see only personnel *not* involved in contemplated administrative action, (but what of the person in need of help who is also in administrative difficulty)? Should he see whoever is administratively referred but refrain from any diagnosis or recommendation? Should he see whoever is referred and make only diagnoses and recommendations that will be construed as being in the best interests of the employee? (Then his silences will be understood as a negative report!) Should he see whoever is referred and make a medical psychiatric diagnosis without recommendation? . . .

Dr. Hartog believes that the agency consultant must accept medical responsibility for diagnosis and treatment or referral; in the process he must either respect confidential communications or inform the patient that he is not in a position to respect confidences. He must respond to administrative pressure to expedite administrative inclinations by applying "equal counter-pressure to maintain his own professional integrity and the rights of his patient. Eventually administrators learn what are the limits and proper role of the psychiatrist."

But Hippocrates was less optimistic about what an individual can accomplish in his lifetime: "Life is short and the art long" is one of his aphorisms. Whether doctors can wait until administrators have learned these limits—and whether doctors themselves have given much thought to the limits and the proper role of the doctor in relation to his patient —is doubtful. The individual approach, where each doctor works out for himself the proper role he is to play, giving weight to both the ideal doctor-patient relationship and such necessities of modern life as hiring, firing, and insurance, demands from the doctor strength of mind and a sophisticated understanding of civil liberties and rights of patients. Whether the good will and good offices of the individual physician are enough, or whether new codes of ethical behavior should be formulated to deal with the new roles of the nontreating and salaried physicians, is a topic for debate and, one hopes, for agreement.

Doctor and Patient:
Confidentiality and Privilege

MOST LAYMEN, even most psychiatrists, assume that whatever a patient says in the course of treatment is a privileged communication that the doctor cannot be required to repeat on the witness stand, and that a privileged communication is one that the law requires to be kept secret. Both assumptions are incorrect.

Whether communications are privileged varies from jurisdiction to jurisdiction: the patient does not have the same right that a lawyer's client has to prevent the disclosure of confidences. Moreover, the privilege that is sometimes given by the law applies to only the courtroom or testimonial situation.

ETHICAL OBLIGATION

No one would deny that the physician has an ethical obligation to hold confidential much of the material divulged to him by patients or discovered as a result of the examination of patients. The doctor-patient relationship—like the minister-parishioner and lawyer-client relationships—depends on complete honesty, mutual trust, and an atmosphere in which patients can disclose all their concerns.

The Hippocratic Oath embodies this ethical concept: "That whatsoever I shall see or hear of the lives of men which is not fitting to be spoken, I will keep inviolably secret."[1] *The Principles of Medical Ethics*, issued by the Judicial Council for the American Medical Association, state:

A physician may not reveal the confidences entrusted to him in the course of medical attendance, or the deficiencies he may observe in the character of patients, unless he is required to do so by law or unless it becomes necessary in order to protect the welfare of the individual or of the community.[2]

And confidentiality was originally a matter for the physician's conscience.

Against disclosures outside the courtroom the legislatures have provided no protection. So far as statutes go, the doctor may with legal impunity chat

222

about the case at a cocktail party or describe it in detail in a medical journal. Legal protection here is afforded only insofar as the courts might find an invasion of the right of privacy, and recovery on this ground will be allowed only if the publication went beyond the limits of reasonableness and decency.[3]

In 22 states, statutes provide that willful betrayal of a professional secret is grounds for revocation of a medical license. But few cases have been brought under these statutes, and Stetler and Moritz state that these statutes "do not seem to be well known."[4] A physician does have civil liability for damages directly caused by the violation of a confidence, but few cases deal directly with this issue, indicating that this protection against unauthorized disclosures is rarely invoked.

LEGAL DEVELOPMENT

Although the tradition of confidentiality on the part of the physician goes back to Hippocrates, the legal development has concerned not confidentiality as much as privilege—the right of a party at law to have certain testimony kept out of the trial proceeding.

Originally, under English common law, there had been no compulsion to testify; certain categories of people considered unreliable—because of religion, sex, infancy, condition of servitude, interest in the outcome of the trial, mental illness, and previous conviction of crime—were held incompetent to testify, and others could testify or not as they chose. In time, most of the grounds of absolute incompetency were eliminated, and the courts allowed these witnesses but reserved the question of their credibility for judicial and jury determination.[5]

In 1562, the policy of testimonial compulsion became the law of England, with a penalty of £10 plus damages for the aggrieved party if a witness refused to testify. DeWitt describes the development of the privilege of not testifying since that time.[6]

Shortly after the policy of testimonial compulsion became established in England, the courts occasionally were confronted by witnesses who refused to answer particular questions put to them on the ground that their testimony would necessarily result in the disclosure of confidential communications or information which, for reasons of public policy or personal honor, they ought not to be compelled to reveal. Usually it was claimed by such witnesses that matters of a genuinely confidential character were not the proper subject of inquiry in courts of law; that, to improve the administration of justice, all persons should be encouraged to come forward with their evidence by shielding them as far as possible from compulsory disclosure of matters strictly confidential. On the other hand, it was urged that the courts were duty bound to see that complete justice was done; that to achieve this objective, no barrier should be erected against the discovery of the truth; that, therefore, no witness should have the right to withhold relevant evidence and thus suppress or conceal the truth, or any portion thereof, no matter how harmful to himself or to others its effect might be, provided it did not tend to convict him of a crime, or subject him to a penalty.

Ultimately, however, the courts became persuaded that the duty of testifying, so onerous at times yet so necessary to the administration of justice, should properly be subject to mitigation in exceptional circumstances. . . . Broadly speaking, the matters affected by the doctrine of privilege may be classified as political, judicial, social, and professional. The more widely known of these privileges are those which relate to state secrets, political votes, trade secrets, religious beliefs, antimarital facts, and self-incriminating matters; those which have been extended to persons standing in a confidential relationship such as husband and wife, grand jurors, petit jurors, judges, arbitrators, public officers, and informers who furnish government officials evidence of crime; and that which is granted to attorneys acting in a professional capacity.

The oldest and least challenged privilege is that accorded to lawyer and client. Says DeWitt: "It appears to be everywhere conceded that the purpose of the privilege is to encourage the employment of professional advisers by persons in need of their services and to promote absolute freedom of consultation by removing all fear on the part of the client that his attorney may be compelled to disclose in court the communications made to, or the information acquired by, him in the course of his professional employment."[7]

Under common law, at least for the last several hundred years, communications to clergymen or other ecclesiastical officers are not considered privileged, but modern judges have been reluctant to force disclosure. However, if the clergyman volunteers to testify, some judges have accepted testimony in spite of the objections of the "penitent" (this type of relationship is known in law as the priest-penitent relationship). In 37 states and three territories of the United States, the common law policy has been changed by statutes, most of which provide that a minister of the gospel or a priest of any denomination is incompetent to testify concerning communications made to him in his professional character, in the course of discipline enjoined by the rules of practice of his denomination. The armed services in their court-martial provisions also recognize the privilege.[8] These statutes, rather than enlarging the common-law rule, by turning a custom into a right have narrowed it, because the tendency of courts has been towards strict construction of the statutes. Unless the penitent's statements to the minister were made to him in his professional character and in the course of church duties ordered by the rules of the religious denomination, and unless they are penitential in character or made in obedience to religious duty, the privilege does not exist.

A Methodist minister was permitted to testify in an Arkansas wills case that he had had conversations with the testator in which he spoke of his adulterous relationship with his housekeeper, been penitent about his conduct, and expressed a desire to join the church. The testimony was held not privileged; the court said it did not appear that the statements made to the minister were in his professional capacity, nor was there testimony that this was in course of discipline enjoined by rules of practice of the religious denomination.[9] In a Kentucky murder prosecution, another Methodist minister testified that when he had visited the defendant in jail, the defendant had admitted guilt to him. The court said that the visit of the pastor to the jail was voluntary and unsolicited, that the statement was not made because of a religious duty, and that the statement was not shown to be penitential, made to the minister in his professional capacity and in pursuance of Methodist rules of practice. Again, the privilege was not allowed.[10]

On the other hand, in *Mullen* vs *United States*,[11] confessions made to a Lutheran minister, by a nonchurch member to whom he had promised spiritual aid if she confessed, were ruled privileged. Carolyn Mullen had left her children chained in her home while she was absent. The minister testified for Mrs. Mullen as a character witness. After his testimony, she took the stand and denied chaining the children. The minister then asked to see the trial judge in chambers, revealed that Mrs. Mullen had confessed chaining the children, and was recalled to the stand to give this testimony. The United States Court of Appeals reversed the subsequent conviction, acting under the authority of Rule 26 of the Federal Rules of Criminal Procedure, which states that the privileges of witness shall be governed in federal courts by the principles of the common law as they may be interpreted by the courts in the light of reason and experience. Said the court: "It is true that the trend of decisions has been chiefly in the direction of enlarging rather than restricting the area of admissibility of evidence, but the governing principle is the same. When reason and experience call for recognition of a privilege which has the effect of restricting evidence the dead hand of the common law will not restrain such recognition."

William Harold Tiemann, a Presbyterian minister, in *The Right to Silence*, states that "it seems fair to draw the following conclusions about privileged communications to clergymen under statute law."

Although the statues are often strictly construed, where a statement is made to a clergyman in his professional character, in the course of discipline enjoined by the rules or practice of the religious body to which he belongs, that communication is considered privileged. The clergyman does not have to belong to a denomination which considers confession mandatory, nor does the communication have to consist of a strict confession of sin. Where practice of his denomination encourages a minister to serve as confidant and counselor to his parishioners and where they share with him in confidence their problems, their marital difficulties, and their sins of commission and omission, such communications are generally recognized as privileged.[12]

The communication to lawyer was privileged at common law and the communication to minister, while not privileged, has been—to the degree indicated above—recognized by custom and by statute. Confidential communications between patient and physician were not privileged from disclosure at common law.[13] The European tradition, governed by Civil Law, was different. "Under the Civil Law, communications between a physician and his patient were at all times considered confidential and sacred. Without the consent of the patient, the physician could not disclose at any time, either in court or elsewhere, any information regarding the health or physical condition of the patient which he acquired in his professional capacity. Today, in most European countries, the relationship of physician and patient is completely protected by a cloak of privilege."[14]

Not so in English law. Said Lord Mansfield in 1776, formalizing the common law rule that denies privilege to physicians, contrary to European practice: "If a surgeon was voluntarily to reveal these secrets, to be sure he would be guilty of a breach of honour, and of great indiscretion; but, to give that information in a court of justice, which by law of the land he is bound to do, will never be imputed to him as any indiscretion whatever."[15] The common law, which is the law in England, most of the British Commonwealth, and of American jurisdictions in the absence of statutes to the contrary, not only does not give this privileged status to communications to physicians, but has gone so far as to order a physician to disclose information in the face of explicit governmental regulations against disclosure. In a 1920 English case, *Garner* vs *Garner*,[16] divorce was sought on the grounds of adultery and cruelty. The cruelty alleged was communication of syphilis by husband to wife. Dr. K. was called to prove plaintiff had incurred syphilis; he declined to testify on the ground that the Venereal Diseases Regulations absolutely prohibited him from disclosing information acquired while serving at a venereal disease clinic. The court ordered him to make the disclosure and held that the Regulations could not override the general law of England, which requires a physician to disclose the health of the patient whenever that is relevant to the issue before the court. This case has been called "the high water mark" in the application of the common law rule.

New York was the first state to pass a physician-patient privileged communication law, in 1828. The philosophy that prompted it cannot be known, but it is surmised that it was intended to encourage the utmost confidence between the patient and doctor, so that all symptoms would be brought forth and the doctor would be in a position to make a correct diagnosis. Probably the need to feel certain that communications would be respected concerning venereal conditions, which frequently are involved in legal cases where privilege has been involved, was an important factor in the passage of the legislation.

Most early statutes, all modeled after the New York law, were couched in general terms, and they produced results not contemplated by the legislators.

It soon became evident that the statutes prevented the testimony of physicians in probate and testamentary proceedings, hospitalization for mental illness, determinations of incompetency, personal injury cases, and actions by physicians for services rendered. In addition, these early laws failed to provide any method of waiver by the patient or someone representing him. The privilege laws, instead of offering the patient protection against the disclosure of confidential information, prohibited the disclosure of any information about the patient's condition regardless of its benefit to the patient or his willingness to have it disclosed.[17]

At present, 36 states have privilege laws, and these vary widely in scope, wording, and limitations. In Wisconsin, for example, privilege does not apply to cases involving homicide, mental competency, and suits brought against the physician. In New Mexico, the privilege is restricted to the physician's knowledge of "venereal or loathsome diseases." In North Carolina, a judge of a superior court may compel disclosure if "in his opinion it is necessary to the administration of justice." In contrast to the early New York statute but in conformity with common law practice, it is now clearly established that the privilege belongs not to the doctor but to the patient: if the patient waives the privilege, the doctor is free to testify; if the patient does not waive the privilege and an appropriate statute exists, the physician can only testify to the two facts that he is a physician and did treat the patient. He is then excused from the stand.

The privilege has been narrowly confined. Nurses and medical assistants are included in only a few statutes, and dentists, druggists, medical students, and Christian Science practitioners have been held to be outside the privileged relationship. Says Friedman: "In fact, in some states it is even questionable whether the privilege applies to psychiatrists or psychologists as several statutes are expressly inapplicable to the treatment of mental and emotional disorders."[18] However, in Illinois, despite the fact that, in the absence of statute, common law prevailed, psychiatrist Dr. Roy Grinker, who refused to testify to matters told to him in professional confidence by a patient, was allowed by the court[19] to maintain this refusal.

Customarily, when a psychiatrist's patient expresses fears that what he says will not be held confidential, the psychiatrist will reassure him of the confidentiality of the information and add, perhaps, that even courts of law would not require any such information to be divulged. The psychiatrist would be wrong on two counts. Not all psychiatrists keep information confidential. Although confidentiality is more important in the psychiatrist-patient relationship than in any other doctor-patient relationship, psychiatrists feel free to breach confidentiality in an emergency—such as when a patient confides he plans to commit suicide; and often they are forced to breach confidentiality when they have to deal with a third person—such as a court that requires the patient to present himself for treatment, or a relative who is paying the therapy bills and wants an occasional progress report. The extent to which any doctor responds to requests for information depends on his personal ethics as well as his evaluation of the situation.

The psychiatrist's reassurance that courts do not require divulgence is equally erroneous. In a 1958 Utah case, a physician in another state in the interest of a local girl wrote to a psychiatrist in Utah for information—desired by the parents of the girl—about a former patient with whom she was keeping company. The Utah physician supplied this information although he had not had the young man as a patient for a period of seven years.[20] The patient brought a libel suit against his former physician, alleging that the letter contained false and derogatory information acquired in connection with treatment for a mental disorder. The Utah supreme court stated that a physician's responsibility to keep a confidence may be outweighed by a higher duty to supply information under certain circumstances and that this duty may extend to the protection of third persons. Furthermore, it did not disagree with the trial court's finding that protecting the happiness of the young girl was sufficient reason to justify the disclosure. The Court stated that if four criteria are met—good faith, fair reporting, conveying only such information as necessary to accomplish the purpose of protecting the third party, and giving information only to persons necessary to accomplish the purpose of protection—then such information can be given.

This case, *Berry* vs *Moench*, is particularly interesting because it demonstrates how far a doctor can go in revealing confidential information, attempting to thwart the plans of his former patient, misrepresenting the facts of the former doctor-patient relationship and in general departing from the Hippocratic injunction to keep information "inviolably secret" without incurring legal liability. In 1949 Berry was having marital difficulties and at his wife's request saw Dr. Moench who diagnosed him as a psychopathic personality with a manic depressive depression and gave him four electroshock treatments. He never saw Dr. Moench again. Seven years later he was living in another state , was divorced, and was keeping company with the girl whose parents initiated the query to Dr. Moench.

Dr. Moench's reply began with a quick nod to the concept of confidentiality: "Since I do not have his authorization, the patient you mentioned in your last letter will remain nameless." Then the doctor got down to business.

> He was treated here in 1949 as an emergency. Our diagnosis was manic depressive depression in a psychopathic personality. . . .
> He had one brother as a manic, and his father committed suicide. . . .
> The patient was attempting to go through school on the G.I. bill. . . . Instead of attending class he would spend most of the days and nights playing cards for money.
> Because of family circumstances, we treated him for a mere token charge (and I notice even that has never been paid).
> During his care here, he purchased a brand new Packard, without even money to buy gasoline.
> He was in constant trouble with the authorities during the war. . . .
> . . . did not do well in school, and never did really support his wife and children.
> Since he was here, we have repeated requests for his record indicating repeated trouble. . . .
> My suggestion to the infatuated girl would be to run as fast and as far as she possibly could in any direction away from him.
> Of course if he doesn't marry her, he will marry someone else and make life hell for that person. The usual story is repeated unsuccessful marriages and a trail of tragedy behind.

In spite of this letter, the marriage took place; the bride's parents disowned their daughter. At the trial Dr. Moench admitted that some of the derogatory information he passed on came from the original referring doctor, some from Berry, some from his former wife and former sister-in-law and he was unable seven years later to recall what information came from what sources. The court noted: "Experience teaches that the unhappy wife of a blighted marriage is not really the most impartial source of information as to the conduct and character of a disappointing husband; less so a sister-in-law. Dr. Moench admitted relying on their statements." The court also noted that in contrast to the picture of him drawn by Dr. Moench, Berry testified that he had been in the top 1% of his class in high school, had been editor-in-chief of the school paper, had done above average work in college. He testified that far from being penniless when he bought his car, he had money in the bank plus a $4,000 inheritance. Concerning the bill, all but $5 had been paid. (He did admit to failing two college courses and to some minor troubles with authorities.) In spite of the doctor's reliance on hearsay, his failure to identify the sources of his derogatory information, his seven-year-long lack of contact with the patient, and the breach of confidentiality, the court rules that such considerations were outweighed by the doctor's duty to "protect the happiness" of the young girl.

Although it is sometimes said that a physician incurs civil liability for unauthorized disclosure of information outside the legal setting, courts are often reluctant to penalize the physician if his disclosure was motivated by some reason other than malice. In the classic *Simonsen* vs *Swenson*,[21] a physician diagnosed his patient's disease as syphilis but told him he could not be sure until a Wassermann test was done. Feeling that the disease was highly contagious, he advised the patient to move out of the hotel in which he lived. When the patient did not move, the physician told the hotel proprietor, who ordered the patient to move. The Wassermann proved negative. The court said that a wrongful breach of confidence would give rise to a civil action for damages, but that here the physician had a duty to disclose his suspicions to prevent the spread of disease.

PSYCHIATRY AND CONFIDENTIALITY

The Group for the Advancement of Psychiatry has emphasized the special requirement in psychiatry for the maintenance of confidentiality.[22]

Among physicians, the psychiatrist has a special need to maintain confidentiality. His capacity to help his patients is completely dependent upon their willingness and ability to talk freely. This makes it difficult if not impossible for him to function without being able to assure his patients of confidentiality and, indeed, privileged communication. . . . There is wide agreement that confidentiality is a *sine qua non* for successful psychiatric treatment. The relationship may well be likened to that of the priest-penitent or the lawyer-client. Psychiatrists not only explore the very depths of their patients' conscious, but their unconscious feelings and attitudes as well. Therapeutic effectiveness necessitates going beyond a patient's awareness and, in order to do this, it must be possible to communicate freely. A threat to secrecy blocks successful treatment.

Obviously this statement refers not to the organic psychiatrists who rely on medication, but to the psychoanalytically oriented therapists. The basic concepts—the existence of an unconscious, the expression of conflicts that have an unconscious component as a symptom, the structure of the psychic apparatus—are derived from Freud and so, too, is the method of treatment. Although most dynamic psychiatrists are not psychoanalysts, the psychoanalytic method has dominated most modern schools of psychiatry. One of Freud's main technics, use of a couch so the patient will not see the analyst's face, is used primarily by psychoanalysts and psychiatrists much influenced by psychoanalysis.

One other Freudian technic is generally used, the invocation of the so-called basic rule, or rule of free association.

In 1899, Freud's first great and most influential work appeared, *The Interpretation of Dreams.* Talking of the procedure of psycho-analysis, he said[23]:

I have been engaged for many years (with a therapeutic aim in view) in unravelling certain psychopathological structures—hysterical phobias, obsessional ideas, and so on. . . . If a pathological idea of this sort can be traced back to the elements in the patient's mental life from which it originated, it simultaneously crumbles away and the patient is freed from it. . . . My patients were pledged to communicate to me every idea or thought that occurred to them in connection with some particular subject. . . .

This involves some psychological preparation of the patient. We must aim at bringing about two changes in him: an increase in the attention he pays to his own psychical perceptions and the elimination of the criticism by which he normally sifts the thoughts that occur to him. In order that he may be able to concentrate his attention on his self-observation it is an advantage for him to lie in a restful attitude and shut his eyes. It is necessary to insist explicitly on his renouncing all criticism of the thoughts that he perceives. We therefore tell him that the success of the psycho-analysis depends on his noticing and reporting whatever comes into his head and not being misled, for instance, into suppressing an idea because it strikes him as unimportant or irelevant or because it seems to him meaningless. He must adopt a completely impartial attitude to what occurs to him. . . .

More recently, Waelder has described the use of the couch and of the basic rule as a necessary part of technic used to achieve the analytic situation, which he defines as "a situation of artificial, partial, and controlled regression for the purpose of a study of inner conflicts."[24]

. . . the analysand is asked to lie down on a couch and to relax; this is a position of defenselessness, similar to the position assumed by patients in medical procedures. The analyst sits behind the analysand; he can see him without being seen. The unilateral exposure is further emphasized by the requirement that the analysand reveal everything about himself in complete frankness—which invariably includes confessing embarrassing things; the analyst does not reciprocate in kind. All this contributes to putting the analysand into a position similar to that of a child vis-a-vis an adult.

In addition to refraining from censoring his thoughts, the analysand goes further: he gives up his usual type of orderly goal-directed speech in favor of speech reflecting the random progression of thought, which Waelder calls "impulse-ridden" expression. This is the so-called basic rule or rule of free association.

The analysand is urged to abandon the ordinary habit of goal-directed thought, and instead to permit everything freely to enter his mind and to verbalize it as soon as it appears, without censorship or editing of any kind.

The (relative) elimination of conscious steering tendencies which determine the ordinary course of organized thought leads neither to a psychologically meaningless jumble of ideas nor to a sequence of association in which each idea stimulates the emergence of others similar to it or connected with it in space or time—as was assumed by the association psychology dominant at the end of the nineteenth century (Wundt)—but rather to a situation in which *unconscious* steering tendencies, ordinarly subdued or obfuscated by the superimposed conscious steering tendencies, are permitted to prevail. Hence the unconscious begins to express itself.[25]

Because Freud was part of the European tradition, with its dependence on Civil Law, he would have had no qualms when he instructed the patient to talk in a completely uncensored fashion. No privileged communication need be invoked in a court of law, since the doctor-patient communication was completely confidential. No reference appears in Freud to the subject of legal privilege. The only problem Freud had in the sphere of patient communications was his own indecision and internal debates concerning his right to publish case histories.

Freud's earliest approach to psychoanalysis, the essay and case studies which represented his collaboration with Josef Breuer in working out a hypnotic and cathartic therapy method, was published in 1895. The foreword to *Studies on Hysteria*,[26] by the joint authors, states that the selection of the case histories "could not unfortunately be determined on purely scientific grounds. Our experience is derived from private practice in an educated and literate social class, and the subject matter with which we deal often touches upon our patients' most intimate lives and histories. It would be a grave breach of confidence to publish material of this kind, with the risk of the patients being recognized and their acquaintances becoming informed of facts which were confided only to the physician. It has therefore been impossible for us to make use of some of the most instructive and convincing of our observations." And when *The Interpretation of Dreams* was written, Freud relied largely on his own dreams as material for the book, although he gave as his reasons not his patients' claim to confidentiality but the fact that the presence of neurotic features in the dreams of his patients made them atypical and undesirable for his purpose.

The founder of psychoanalysis, hampered by the necessity for confidentiality, wrote only five major case histories during his long lifetime. The first of these, *A Case of Hysteria*, was ready for publication in 1901, but Freud could not make up his mind to publish the case history and it finally appeared four years later. The editor of the first journal to which it had been sent declined to publish it, apparently on the grounds that it was a breach of discretion. Of the four other major case histories, one was of a small boy and one was written not about a patient but about the published autobiography of a psychotic judge. The two other histories were described by Freud as having been reported only in a "fragmentary manner."[27]

Psychoanalytic theory and practice eventually spread to the United States and found here its most congenial audience. The influence on psychiatry of psychoanalytic theory has been greater in this country than anywhere else. And wherever Freud's influence has gone, with it has gone the injunction to follow the Basic Rule, to speak randomly about whatever comes into mind in an entirely uncensored way, without fear of consequences.

But possibly the consequences should be feared, for two reasons. First, the psychiatrist pursuing the secret thoughts of the patient is not always in the relationship of doctor-patient to the narrator of the intimate knowledge. The patient may trust the doctor as a psychiatrist; the psychiatrist may not be bound by a relationship to the patient if he is examining at the request of a third party. Second, the confidentiality of the psychiatrist-patient relationship has not been unequivocally recognized by United States courts.

The complications of the situation in which the doctor acts as the agent of a third party have been described in the previous chapter. GAP's Committee on Psychiatry and Law has discussed this problem frankly.[28] Occasionally, a lawyer will employ a psychiatrist to examine a client in his behalf. The psychiatrist examining a patient for a lawyer is fully covered by the lawyer's privilege, since he is an agent for the lawyer, even in those jurisdictions where no medical privilege exists. Sometimes psychiatrists cooperate in a process in which individuals volunteer to be examined by such special technics as "truth serum" or "lie detector tests."

This poses the difficult problem of whether or not the consequences of the waiver, that is, agreeing to undergo such test, may be tantamount to self-incrimination. For, when an individual offers to submit to amytal interviews, projective tests, or psychiatric interviews, he cannot 'know' in advance what he waives. On the other hand, if he is informed of what emerged through the use of such techniques, he would then be in a position to decide whether to exercise his right of privilege. Questions with respect to admissibility of such evidence must be settled by the court. In jurisdictions where there is no waiver because there is no privilege, there is a basic policy question of whether enough would be gained by the admission of such data, to offset the potential risks of 'involuntary' loss of privacy, 'involuntary' self-incrimination, or declaration against self-interest.[29]

The GAP report also notes that with the general growth of industrial medicine, large companies have retained psychiatrists to care for their employees' emotional problems. "If the psychiatrist is administratively tied to the personnel division of a company, the confidential relationship cannot exist, and it behooves him to clarify his position with the employee. We regard failure to do so as a serious abridgement of the physician's ethical responsibility."

This report devotes special attention to the psychiatrist working for public mental hospitals, prisons, and law enforcement agencies.[30]

The psychiatrist is called upon to serve in two roles: first in the role of therapist, and second, as an agent of the administration of the institution which he serves. Patients in mental hospitals are there as the result of voluntary or involuntary commitment. This process has legal force, and causes many alterations in the patient's life situation. The decision to continue hospitalization may be administrative as well as medical. It is at this point that the roles of the therapist and agent may coincide. While this is socially necessary for many reasons, patients see this alteration of the traditional doctor-patient relationship as placing the therapist in the position of a judge, who may manipulate the patient's future, without the patient's agreement. We emphasize that this departure from the ideal of confidentiality complicates therapy.

In the prison the psychiatrist's function as an agent forces him to juggle an inherently ambiguous situation. His patients identify him with the involuntary, punitive confinement, and he is constantly pressed by the administration to ally himself with the penal function of the institution. We can conceive of the possibility of utilizing a psychiatrist to improve the administration of a prison. However, if he elects this role he must anticipate a proportional decrease of his effectiveness in doctor-patient relationships. When he functions as a therapist, he must adhere to his confidential relationship with the prisoner. Within the prison setting, the psychiatrist who does therapy must find a way to minimize the prisoners' tendency to identify him with the prison authorities.

Special problems confront the psychiatrist in the law enforcement setting, as noted previously. A psychiatrist may be a psychiatrist in name only, acting in fact as an 'inquisitor.' A spurious confidentiality gained by deceit, serves the purpose of transcending the conventional methods of seeking to establish guilt by confessions. We deplore this practice as an open breach of the physician's ethical obligations and we can find no justification for such participation by a psychiatrist.

VERNON MITCHELL AND DR. SCHILT

In September 1960 two employees of the National Security Agency, Vernon Mitchell and William Martin, defected to the USSR. Mitchell had been referred by his physician to a psychiatrist practicing in a Maryland suburb of Washington, D. C., and had been seen for three one-hour interviews. During these interviews, he had discussed his homosexuality, family quarrels and jealousies, and his atheism; he had not disclosed his plan to defect and he had never even mentioned Martin. After the patient had left the country, the psychiatrist, Dr. Clarence Schilt, was subpoenaed by the House Un-American Activities

Committee and gave testimony in a secret session. No evidence was made public whether this testimony was given freely or under pressure. Dr. Schilt refused to divulge his testimony to the press, but, as inevitably happens in Congressional secret proceedings, details of his statement concerning his patient's homosexuality, family problems, and religious feelings were leaked to the press. There was immediate protest in the Washington medical community; in a letter to the *Washington Post*, the Council of the Washington Psychiatric Society stated that it viewed with grave concern "any breach of confidentiality in the doctor-patient relationship" and that this particular breach "may have given rise to apprehension in the minds of psychiatric patients or those contemplating such treatment. Our Council wishes to reassert this principle as binding upon physicians and to deplore departure from this principle. Without the assurance of confidentiality, medical treatment,and especially psychiatric treatment, would be impossible. . . ."[31]

Dr. Schilt practiced in Maryland, and 37 internists and psychiatrists signed a petition to the Medical and Chirurgical Faculty of the State of Maryland requesting an investigation of this "possible breach of medical ethics. Information given to a physician within the doctor-patient relationship," they asserted, "must be considered confidential and must not be disclosed except with the permission of the patient or under certain well-defined criminal circumstances."[32] The Faculty's Professional Conduct Committee ruled in favor of the testifying doctor.

It is the considered opinion of this Committee that Dr. Schilt did not violate the law of Maryland, and that the interests of the nation transcend those of the individual. In addition, the Committee was informed that the testimony of Dr. Schilt was given in secret session to the House Un-American Activities Committee and its public release was through this Committee rather than through Dr. Schilt. The Committee feels that Dr. Schilt acted in an ethical and cooperative manner with public authorities on this matter.[33]

Two eminent authorities on the subject give apparently contrasting views on this incident. Dr. Zigmond Lebensohn, in a signed editorial in the *Journal of the American Medical Association*,[34] although emphasizing the absolute essentiality of confidentiality to the practice of psychotherapy, also noted that "it is important to remember that the patient's confidences cannot be protected in a legal proceeding unless the right is granted by state law." Dr. Victor Sidel, in the *New England Journal of Medicine*,[35] stresses the irrelevance of the fact that Dr. Schilt did not violate the law of Maryland (which state has no law of privileged doctor-patient communication) to the greater problem of a physician's ethical, professional responsibility to his patient.

Sidel feels that changes in the *Principles of Ethics* of the American Medical Association have shifted, in a decade, from an emphasis on the doctor's professional role ("medicine . . . knows nothing of national enmities") to the emphasis on the doctor's role as a citizen "on whose shoulders the destiny of our nation rests." He also notes the change in the "American" ethics concerning confidentiality: *from* "confidences . . . should never be revealed except when imperatively required by the laws of the state" (or in a case of communicable disease) *to* the injunction against the revelation of confidences "unless he is required to do so by law or unless it becomes necessary in order to protect the welfare of the individual or of the community."

At the same time that the needs to serve the community were receiving additional emphasis in American medicine, members of both the European and the American medical professions, acting through the World Medical Association, were formulating a code of ethical principles—a "modern language version" of the Hippocratic Oath—called the Oath of Geneva, which pledges without reservation that "I will hold in confidence all that my patient confides in me." This was adopted by the WMA in 1948, and the following year in its International Code of Medical Ethics the same group stated: "A doctor owes to his patient absolute secrecy on all which has been confided to him or which he knows because of the confidence entrusted to him. . . ." In 1954, an interpretative statement concerning this section said: "Professional secrecy by its very nature must be absolute. It must be observed in all cases ('ergo omnes'). A secret which is shared is no longer a secret. Exceptions to the rule of professional secrecy can be made only in special cases such as reporting the incidence of epidemic or communicable diseases." Thus, says Sidel, "one sees a striking difference between the trend in published ethics in international medicine and that in American medicine."

Since the publication of Sidel's article, the WMA has taken another step to strengthen its stand on confidentiality. In 1965, during its 19th assembly, held in London, it unanimously adopted a resolution stating that physicians, like lawyers, should be privileged witnesses in court cases in all countries and should not be compelled to divulge secrets about patients.[36] Dr. Derek Stevenson, secretary of the British Medical Association, which sponsored the resolution, said that his group feels "that the time has come—if it is not already past—that national legislatures be asked to recognize this fundamental principle, the obligation of medical secrecy. Exceptions are inevitable but should be limited in number and made only in consultation with the medical association of the country concerned."

Dr. Stevenson said that the British group's statement of policy allows doctors to divulge information required by statute, as in reporting infectious diseases, or in cases where the patient's own welfare requires disclosure.

The Group for the Advancement of Psychiatry has said that the special character of psychiatric treatment requires confidentiality as a *sine qua non* for successful therapy and so has recommended the safeguarding of the doctor-patient relationship by laws in all United States jurisdictions to give communications to psychiatrists in the course of treatment unqualified privilege, placing them on the same basis as privileged communications between attorney and client.[37]

DR. GRINKER AND JUDGE FISHER

Very possibly, not additional legislation but the courage of the testifying psychiatrist is the answer to the problem of lack of privilege. In 1952, Dr. Roy Grinker, noted Chicago psychiatrist, was called as a witness in the suit for alienation of affections brought by a husband against another man.[38] Since he had been the wife's therapist, Dr. Grinker was in a position to know the truth or falsity of the charges, but he refused to divulge in court confidences, possibly prejudicial to her, that the patient had communicated to him.   Dr. Grinker expressed his willingness to be cited for contempt of court, if necessary, and to take the issue to the appellate court.   The trial court ruled, however, that a psychiatrist is not required to testify to such confidential communications, even in the absence of any Illinois statute giving privilege to the doctor-patient relation, because the psychiatrist-patient relationship is more deserving of privilege than the ordinary doctor-patient relationship, said Judge Fisher.   The relationship is "unique and not at all similar to the relationship between physician and patient."   Zenoff has minimized the effect of this decision.[39]   "Since the courts have universally held that the privilege can be created by statute only, however, the decision in *Binder* vs *Ruvell* would probably have been reversed if the case had been appealed."   GAP has also denied much legal significance to this case, on the basis that the case established no precedent because it was never appealed.[40]   Certainly, however, the case does represent a precedent in its own jurisdiction and certainly, as the GAP report concedes, "it has been influential."   Perhaps the reason that this problem has not come before the courts more frequently than it has since 1952 is the strong decision of Judge Fisher in support of the strong stand of Dr. Grinker.

RECORDS AND REPORTS

Despite the fact that common law does not protect the relationship of psychiatrist and patient and that statutes that confer a privilege in this area can be construed narrowly, it is hard to imagine an unbiased court that would not accord at least as much status to psychiatric confidences—in the light of the need for confidentiality in the dynamic psychiatric relationship—as it gives to lawyer and client without reservation, and as it tends to honor, without strictly giving, in the priest and penitent relationship. The problems here relate primarily not to privilege but to the ethical concept of confidentiality, and they center not on court proceedings but on such complicated issues in modern life as hospital and military records, reports to insurance companies, obligations to a third-party employer. For instance, privilege has never been secured for military personnel in psychiatric treatment; psychiatrists and records may be ordered to appear before a courts-martial, although chaplains can assert the privilege.

The New York State Supreme Court recently ruled that a physician was justified in disclosing to the Air Force that his patient's absences from his work as a civilian employee were due to alcoholism, despite the patient's unwillingness to have this information supplied.[41] The physician, in his successful defense of a suit for damages, claimed that he had an overriding duty to make the disclosure when requested to do so by a military unit of the government. One commentator notes that with more than two million civilian Federal employees who are the patients of private practitioners, the results of this case make the physician's decision as to when a protected confidence remains so "even more difficult to determine."

On the celebration of the Centenary of the Mexican National Academy of Medicine, Dr. Ignacio Chávez spoke of "Professional Ethics in Medicine in Our Time."[42] Reviewing the periods when doctors tried to observe absolute secrecy and the later periods when the law placed restrictions on secrecy, notably in reporting criminal acts and some contagious diseases, he spoke of the new problems of medical ethics that have appeared in the wake of the socialization of medicine and are still unsolved. Of the Mexican National Social Security, he said that "in order to give help in case of sickness, to pay indemnizations, disablement premiums, life insurance, etc., requires complete and accurate information from the doctors. It requires detailed reports covering everything, including hereditary or family illness, which the patients are very reluctant to mention if there is a case of madness or epilepsy, pathological antecedents, although they may include syphilis, pregnancy or abortions, and of course a complete report of the present illness, including analyses, radiographs, and laboratory data."

Professional secrecy has been torn to pieces. The National Social Security has its reasons, and they are good ones for wanting to know everything, because without strict control they could not accept such a large financial commitment.

The patient also has good reasons for not wanting to reveal all his secrets, nor have them passed from hand to hand by all the employees in all the various offices through which his case history must pass before assistance can be authorized. And between the two extremes stands the doctor, urged by one side to reveal, and by the other side to conceal.

INFORMAL RELATIONSHIPS

Perhaps the most frequent and possibly the most important site of abuse of confidentiality is in a doctor's informal relationships with friends, neighbors, colleagues, and wife. Says GAP, "Doctors as a group tend to talk shop, even in social situations where there is a great risk of jeopardizing confidentiality. Psychiatrists are no exception. In social settings psychiatric 'gossip' about patients is to be condemned and constitutes a direct violation of the ethical responsibilities."[43]

PSYCHOLOGISTS AND OTHERS

Psychologists, although they may do the same type of treatment as a psychiatrist, and the few psychoanalysts who are not medical doctors are clearly not within the scope of any doctor-patient privilege. The legislatures of nine states have given the psychologist a special testimonial privilege.[44] That a psychologist has been given this privilege while a psychiatrist has not, specifically, probably is not evidence —as some commentators have assumed—that psychologists are more highly regarded than psychiatrists. But it is evidence that state legislators act on the presumption that psychiatrists are better protected by law and custom in this area than psychologists and other therapists, even in the absence of appropriate statutes.

In the years to come, psychiatric services will be increasingly desired: the shortage of psychiatrists will become more acute. More and more, psychologists, social workers, and nurses will be utilized for therapy. In time, the needs of the patient with emotional problems for the protection of a confidential relationship—whether with a doctor or a nondoctor—must be clarified in the courts and the legislatures if this type of therapy is seen as valuable and worthy of development.

CURRENTS AND CROSS-CURRENTS

These questions and the larger questions of the shape of medicine and the shape of society stir in the consciousness of thoughtful men. A medical writer, Michael J. O'Neill, has described some summer thoughts, while sailing with his wife and children in a small sloop, on the contrast between simplicity and organization[45]:

Here we were, one of the smallest units of society, a husband, wife, and three children, sailing across Nantucket Sound, self-contained, content, free of complexity. Why did our usual life have to be different? Why must privacy and freedom drown in confusion over the organization of modern society? For one of the great issues of our time . . . is whether privacy, individuality, and personal self-respect can be preserved in the face of growing social complexity. Or must these values be sacrificed still further for efficiency and equal opportunity?

In other years, a doctor and his patient could achieve complete privacy. They met alone in office or home, both sufficient to each other. All that either needed was in the doctor's head or a small leather bag. But now there are constant intruders—hospitals and specialists, machines and technicians, insurance carriers and employers and unions. Solo practice is giving way to team care; government is coming in as a third party. The treatment is more sophisticated, more efficient, perhaps, but the old privacy is gone. And this subtracts something from life.

Our exploding population—most dramatic in the Negro ghettos of the big cities—is producing its own gross distortions. As more and more people are jammed together, their privacy and their individuality are compromised. And this demands more social organization and more government action. . . .

There are currents and crosscurrents. While increasing government involvement in health care tends to stimulate the depersonalization of medicine for those who can afford to pay, it may mean more dignity and independence for the needy. But the over-all trend is toward less privacy and individuality as our society is ever more highly organized to meet its increasingly complex problems.

These are one man's thoughts as he contrasts the solitude and escape that are possible only to the self-contained with the organization and the complexity that grow in our urban civilization.

One cannot help yearning for the boat and the open sea again, for the simpler life. Unfortunately, a boat must eventually return to port—and reality.

Epilogue: Pursuit of Agreement

WE HAVE SAID that law is absolute and seeks for absolute answers. It sets down precedents, which can be applied to similar situations. Psychiatry, on the other hand, is relativistic. Psychiatrists find it hard to define what is "right" and what is "wrong"; they see emotional factors that pull a man in different directions, with a choice to be made that under some circumstances could be right and under others wrong—with never a chance to run a controlled experiment to let him know what the result of the other choice would have been.

Although not denying the value of precedents, psychiatry reserves the right to make a fresh determination in every case, because—unlike law, which stresses similarities—psychiatry stresses differences: this robber is different from other robbers because his parents were divorced when he was two and his mother was promiscuous.

The area where law and psychiatry approach each other represents debatable ground, but the opposing forces that battle on this ground are sometimes hard to identify. The lawyer can be characterized as more interested in laws than in people, but he may be defending the rights and liberties of a committed patient, while the doctor, theoretically more interested in the patient's own welfare, would summarily lock him up for treatment.

The areas of disagreement remain, but they decrease in size as each side learns to respect the position of the other. At one time, lawyers had little use for psychiatric testimony, and psychiatrists, on the other hand, were ready to take over the burden of the administration of criminal justice from the courts. During a period when more moderate thinking prevails, it can be seen that two claims can coexist if the claims are less extreme. The lawyer can accept the responsibility of making the final legal determination but still be receptive to the psychiatric concepts that can help him come to fair conclusions. The psychiatrist can recognize that although he cannot be omnipotent, he still has the crucial job of explaining to the courts and to the world the buried motivations and the irrational urges and needs that law would tend to overlook or ignore.

With mutual respect, this understanding can be attained; but it takes time to understand another's point of view. Lawyers are busy and psychiatrists are busy, and it is easier to operate on hunches and wishes than to come to a better understanding of the field of the other and to comprehend a different point of view. Time and energy are limiting factors. Like the vaudevillian with a trick trunk, when we stow away one problem, another pops out. When we solve the problem of infant mortality, we face overpopulation, and when we solve the problem of poverty, we face materialism.

Law and psychiatry command our attention, but there are other concerns, at home and abroad. We face the problems of raising our children, revising society, maintaining peace. It is hard to give the problems of forensic psychiatry the attention they need.

But the task is worth pursuing. Psychiatrists understand better than lawyers that one area of sickness in the individual affects the whole, that a neurosis is not self-contained but makes its presence felt in many areas of the personality. Lawyers understand better than psychiatrists that liberties and rights cannot be abrogated in some areas without affecting all areas. In the midst of world-shaking concerns, the fate of the individual, at least in our society, is still paramount.

Bibliography

THIS BIBLIOGRAPHY gives by chapter, and sometimes comments on, the sources of *PURSUIT OF AGREEMENT: Psychiatry and the Law.*

The most frequent sources will be abbreviated as follows:

Cameron   Cameron, D. E.: Forensic Psychiatry and Child Psychiatry, International Psychiatry Clinics, Boston, Little, Jan, 1965.

Curran   Curran, W. J.: Law and Medicine, Boston, Little, 1960.

Davidson   Davidson, H. A.: Forensic Psychiatry, ed. 2, New York, Ronald, 1965.

Deutsch   Deutsch, A.: The Mentally Ill in America, New York, Columbia Univ Press, 1946.

GAP Report   Group for the Advancement of Psychiatry: Report No. 45, Confidentiality and Privileged Communication in the Practice of Psychiatry, June, 1960.

Guttmacher and Weihofen   Guttmacher, M. S., and Weihofen, H.: Psychiatry and The Law, New York, Norton, 1952.

JAMA   Journal of the American Medical Association.

Long   Long, R. H.: The Physician and the Law, ed. 2, New York, Appleton, 1959.

Med Trib   Medical Tribune.

MWN   Medical World News.

Mod Med   Modern Medicine.

Moritz and Stetler   Moritz, A. R., and Stetler, C. J.: Handbook of Legal Medicine, St. Louis, Mosby, 1964.

Prosser   Prosser, W. L.: Handbook of the Law of Torts, ed. 2, St. Paul, West, 1955.

Report   Lindman, F. T., and McIntyre, D. M., eds.: The Mentally Disabled and the Law, Report of the American Bar Foundation, Chicago, Univ Chicago Press, 1961.

Siegal   Siegal, L. J.: Forensic Medicine, New York, Grune, 1963.

Stetler and Moritz   Stetler, C. J., and Moritz, A. R.: Doctor and Patient and the Law, ed. 4, St. Louis, Mosby, 1962.

Whitlock   Whitlock, F. A.: Criminal Responsibility and Mental Illness, London, Butterworth, 1963.

CHAPTER 1

1. *Lambert* vs *Lambert*, 164 So. 2d 661, 1964.
2. Whitlock: p. 1.
3. Letter of Lewis, Sanford M., MD: Lecturer in Medicine-Law, Rutgers Univ School of Law, to Med Trib, Jan 4, 1963.
4. Whitlock: pp. 2–3.

5. Benet, William Rose (ed.): The Reader's Encyclopedia, New York, Crowell, 1948, p. 281.

CHAPTER 2

1. Opinion of Sir George Jessel in *Printing and Numerical Registering Co.* vs *Sampson*, L. R. 19 Eq. 462 at p. 465, *in* Cheshire, G., and Fifoot, C. H. S.: The Law of Contract, ed. 6, London, Butterworth, 1964, p. 21.
2. Sidgwick, Henry: Elements of Politics (1879), *in* Cheshire and Fifoot, *ibid.*
3. Prosser: p. 14.
4. *Ibid.*: p. 15.
5. Woolf, Virginia: Mrs. Dalloway, New York, Harcourt, A Harvest Book, 1949, p. 149.

CHAPTER 3

1. Lewin, K. K.: A brief psychotherapy method, Penn Med J *68*:43 (#8), 1965.
2. Hodern, A.: Psychiatry: organic approach, J Neuropsychiat *4*:356–365, 1963.
3. Jones, R. O.: *in* Cameron, p. 84.
4. *Ibid.*: p. 87.

CHAPTER 4

1. Letter of Lewis, Sanford M., MD: See ref. 3, chap. 1.
2. *Commonwealth* vs *Woodhouse*, 164 A.2d 98, 1960. The trial is reported in the Harrisburg, Pa, Evening News, May 14, 1957, p. 17, May 15, p. 28, and May 16, p. 17. Although the state had asked for a verdict of first degree murder with a jury recommendation for the electric chair, the verdict was first degree murder without the recommendation for capital punishment. Dr. Woodhouse has been denied an application for parole and is still serving his life sentence.
3. *Both* vs *Nelson*, 202 N.E.2d 494, 1964.
4. *Jenkins* vs *United States*, 307 F.2d 637, 1962. The position of the Amer Psychiat Assn is discussed in its Newsletter, June–Aug, 1962.
5. Rickles, N. K.: The travesty of adversary justice, editorial in Med Trib, Nov 25, 1964, p. 11.
6. Davidson, H. A.: The accountability of the character neurotic, Speech delivered at Arthur P. Noyes Memorial Conf, Norristown State Hosp, Pa, Sep 18, 1965.
7. *Ibid.*
8. Jones, R. O.: *in* Cameron, p. 87.
9. Report: pp. 311–312.

CHAPTER 5

1. *Hotchkiss* vs *National City Bank of New York*, 200 F. 287, 1911.
2. *Woburn National Bank* vs *Woods*, 89 A. 491, 1914.
3. *Raffles* vs *Wichelhaus*, 2 Hurl. & C. 906, 1864.
4. 43 *Corpus Juris Secundum*, Infants §19, Brooklyn, Amer Law Bk Co., pp. 81–82.

5. Report: p. 263.

6. 44 *Corpus Juris Secundum*, Insane Person §98, p. 67.

7. *Ibid.*

8. Cheshire, G., and Fifoot, C. H. S.: The Law of Contract, ed. 6, London, Butterworth, 1964, p. 369.

9. See ref. 6, *supra*.

10. Report: p. 111, footnotes 35–36.

11. NIMH: A draft act governing hospitalization of the mentally ill, Federal Security Agency, Pub Health Serv Pub No. 51, 1952.

12. Report: pp. 111–112.

13. *Ibid.*: p. 112.

CHAPTER 6

1. Report: pp. 198–200, 207–210.

2. *Ibid.*: p. 199.

3. Deutsch: p. 376.

4. Report: p. 199.

CHAPTER 7

1. Report: p. 200.

2. *Ibid.*: p. 200, footnote 19.

3. *Ibid.*: p. 201.

4. *Ibid.*

5. *Ibid.*: Table, p. 211.

6. *Ibid.*: p. 202.

7. *Dribin* vs *Superior Court*, 231 P.2d 809, 812, 1951.

8. Stephens, J., and Astrup, C.: The need for prognostic optimism in schizophrenic illnesses, original article, Psychiat Dig (May), 1965, p. 47 ff.

9. *Ibid.*: Referring to Acta Psychiat Scand Suppl *115*:32, 1957.

10. *Ibid.*: p. 50.

11. Graham, Sheilah, and Frank, Gerold: Beloved Infidel, New York, Holt, 1958, p. 245.

12. Report: pp. 203–204. The two states that permit a mentally ill spouse to sue for divorce are Alabama and Massachusetts.

CHAPTER 8

1. 94 *Corpus Juris Secundum*, Wills §15, p. 691.

2. Report: p. 265.

3. Cox, J. A.: Medical evidence of competency and testamentary capacity, Medicolegal relations, Virginia Law Weekly *Dicta 10*:1958–59, p. 117.

4. *In re Alegria's Estate*, 197 P.2d 571, 1948, cited 94 *CJS*, Wills §17, p. 708.

5. 94 *CJS*, Wills §15, p. 694, fn. 9.

6. Report: pp. 264–265, giving criteria of Page, W. H.: Wills, Cincinnati, Anderson, 1941, *1*:§132, pp. 268–269.

7. Atkinson, T. E.: Handbook of the Law of Wills, ed. 2, St. Paul, West, 1953, p. 243, citing *Fraser* vs *Jennison*, 3 N.W. 882, 900, 1880.

8. *In re Hargrove's Will*, 28 N.Y.S.2d 571, 262 App. Div. 202, affirmed 42 N.E.2d 608, 1942, cited 94 *CJS*, Wills §18, p. 709, fn. 71, and p. 711, fn. 78.

9. *In re Robertson's Estate*, 189 P.2d 615, 1948, cited 94 *CJS*, Wills §18, p. 709, fn. 71.

10. *In re Eveleth's Will*, 157 N.W. 257, 1916, cited Atkinson, ref. 7, *supra*, p. 243, fn. 5.

11. Ray's book went through five editions in his lifetime. The fourth edition, with additions, was published in Boston by Little, Brown in 1860. This was probably the edition familiar to Judge Doe when he wrote the dissenting opinion in *Boardman* vs *Woodman*, see ref. 13, *infra*. The fifth edition, also with additions, was published by Little, Brown in 1871. The 1838 edition, edited by Winfred Overholser, was reprinted in 1962, Cambridge, Belknap Press of Harvard Univ Press.

12. See Reik, L. E.: The Doe-Ray correspondence: a pioneer collaboration in the jurisprudence of mental disease, 63 Yale L.J. 183, 1953.

13. *Boardman* vs *Woodman*, 47 N.H. 120, 1866.

14. Judge Doe's dissent: *in* Curran, p. 640; see also p. 644.

15. Stetler and Moritz: p. 199; Report, pp. 265–266; Stephens, S. J.: Probate psychiatry—examination of testamentary capacity by a psychiatrist as a subscribing witness, 25 Ill. L. Rev. 276–277, 1930.

CHAPTER 9

1. *Boardman* vs *Woodman*, see refs. 11, 13, 14, chap. 8.

2. Biggs, John: The Guilty Mind, New York, Harcourt, 1955, p. 83. For a discussion of *mens rea*, see Roche, P. Q.: The Criminal Mind, New York, Grove, 1958, pp. 82–92.

3. The armor of the law: From the Law-Medicine Institute, Boston Univ, New Eng J Med 270:516–517, 1964. Roche, fn. 2, *supra*, summarizes the M'Naghten philosophy, pp. 89–92.

4. Whitlock: p. 7.

5. Stephen, J. F.: A History of the Criminal Law of England, vol. 2, London, Macmillan, 1883, p. 149.

6. *People* vs *Schmidt*, 110 N.E. 945, 1915.

7. Zilboorg, G.: Misconceptions of legal insanity, Amer J Orthopsychiat 9: 540, 552–553, 1939.

8. Speech by Zilboorg: *in* Guttmacher and Weihofen: p. 406.

9. *United States ex rel. Smith* vs *Baldi*, 192 F.2d 540, 568, 1951.

10. Report: p. 337.

11. *Ibid.*: p. 333.

12. *Durham* vs *United States*, 214 F.2d 862, 1954.

13. Report notes that the *Durham* decision has been rejected by the Court of Military Appeals, by the Fifth and Ninth Circuit Courts of Appeal, and by 13 states: California, Idaho, Illinois, Indiana, Massachusetts, Mississippi, Maryland, Missouri, Nevada, New Jersey, Oklahoma, Vermont, Washington. See Report, p. 341. It has also been rejected by Alaska in *Chase* vs *State*, 369 P.2d 997, 1962; Arizona in *State* vs *Crose*, 357 P.2d 136, 1960; Connecticut in *State* vs *Davies*, 148 A.2d 251, 1959; Delaware in *Longoria* vs *State*, 168 A.2d 695, 1961; Kansas in *State* vs *Andrews*, 357 P.2d 739, 1960; and Pennsylvania in *Commonwealth* vs *Woodhouse*, 164 A.2d 98, 1960. It has been rejected as contrary to existing state statute by Arkansas in *Downs* vs *State*, 330 S.W.2d 281, 1960; Florida, *Piccott* vs *State*, 116 So.2d 626, 1959; Ohio, *State* vs *Robinson*, 168 N.E.2d 328, 1958; and Utah, *State* vs *Poulson*, 381 P.2d 93, 1963. Other cases rejecting *Durham* include Kentucky, *Newsome* vs *Commonwealth*, 366 S.W.2d 174, 1962; and Montana, *State* vs *Noble*, 384 P.2d 504, 1963. Med

Trib, June 5–6, 1965, reports 4 recent cases in states listed above (Arizona, California, Florida, and Maryland) in which higher courts reaffirmed the *M'Naghten* rules. Although the Illinois courts upheld *M'Naghten*, the legislature subsequently by statute adopted the Amer Law Institute Model Penal Code Test, Smith-Hurd Illinois Annotated Statutes, ch. 38 §6–2; Laws 1961, July 28.

14. Although described as a "right or wrong" test, the *M'Naghten* rule (sometimes described in the plural as "rules") has two parts: the accused party at the time the act was committed was "laboring under such a defect of reason, from disease of the mind" as not to know "the nature and quality of the act he was doing, or . . . that he did not know he was doing what was wrong." Report, p. 332, quoting *M'Naghten's Case*, 10 Clark & Fin. 200, 8 Eng. Rep. 718, 1843. If testimony is confined to the narrow issue of ability to distinguish right from wrong, the test can be used to restrict psychiatric testimony; in enlightened jurisdictions and, especially in recent years, consideration of knowing the nature and quality of the act has been used to allow wide scope in psychiatric testimony. For the converse of this (the restriction of psychiatric testimony in a jurisdiction which has substituted a more modern rule for *M'Naghten*), see ref. 28, *infra*.

15. Glueck, S.: Law and Psychiatry: Cold War or *Entente Cordiale*? Baltimore, Johns Hopkins, 1962, p. 10. For a discussion of psychiatric objections to *M'Naghten* and a suggested new approach, see Waelder, R.: Psychiatry and the problem of criminal responsibility, 101 U Pa L Rev 378, 1952.

16. American Law Institute: Model Penal Code, Tent. Draft No. 4, Philadelphia, Amer Law Inst Publishers, 1955, §4.01, p. 27, and comment pp. 156 ff.

17. *Ibid.* This test, with minor changes, is retained in the A.L.I. Model Penal Code Proposed Official Draft, May 4, 1962.

18. *United States* vs *Currens*, 290 F.2d 751, 1961. The 3rd Circuit, a Federal jurisdiction, only deals with criminal matters that are tried in a Federal rather than a state court. In the *Currens* case the Federal court had jurisdiction because a stolen car was taken across state lines.

19. 14 V.I.C. §14(4). See *Government of the Virgin Islands* vs *Smith*, 278 F.2d 169, 1960.

20. *Wion* vs *United States*, 325 F.2d 420, 1963. The New York Times reported on Mar 1, 1966, that the United States Court of Appeals, Second Circuit (which covers New York, Connecticut and Vermont) had unanimously adopted the definition of criminal responsibility of the American Law Institute, rejecting *M'Naghten* as "not in harmony with modern medical science which . . . is opposed to any concept which divides the mind into separate compartments—the intellect, the emotions and the will," pp. 1, 21.

21. Speech: Convention of the Central Neuropsychiat Assn, Med Trib, Nov 16, 1964, p. 31.

22. Burger, W. E.: Psychiatrists, lawyers, and the courts, Fed Probation *28*: 3 (June), 1964.

23. Whitlock: p. 146. On Oct 28, 1965, capital punishment was abolished in Britain. The House of Commons approved the antihanging bill that had first been introduced almost 20 years previously. There had been an unofficial moratorium on hangings since Aug 13, 1964, while Parliament considered the measure. The new law will be reviewed after five years. The Philadelphia Inquirer, Oct 29, 1965, p. 18.

24. Med Trib: June 14, 1965, p. 31.

25. *Ibid.*

26. Sci News Letter: Mar 6, 1965, p. 147; Psychiat Spectator 2:9(#2)Mar, 1965.

27. Brody, E. B.: Psychiatry and the social order, Amer J Psychiat 122:81, 86 (July), 1965.

28. A growing body of decisions indicate that even under a liberal rule such as *Durham*, with a wide scope of psychiatric testimony admitted, decisions can be as harsh as before the change in the law. For one such case, see *State* vs *Park*, 193 A.2d 1, 1963, in which a Maine court's conviction of a 15-year-old boy was upheld.

29. Quoted *in* Williams, Edward Bennett: One Man's Freedom, New York, Atheneum, 1962, p. 247.

CHAPTER 10

1. *Beausoleil* vs *Soeurs de la Charité*, Rapports Judiciaires de Quebec, 1965, B.R., p. 37.

2. Moritz and Stetler: p. 129.

3. *Ibid.*

4. Long: p. 31.

5. *Ibid.*: p. 32.

6. Report: p. 148.

7. Ross, H. A.: Hospitalizing the mentally ill—emergency and temporary commitments, Current Trends in State Legislation 1955–56, Ann Arbor, Univ of Michigan Law School, 1957, p. 534.

8. Med Trib: Feb 13–14, 1965, p. 13.

9. Report: p. 148.

10. 64 Pa. D. & C. 35, 1948.

11. Report: pp. 149–150.

12. *Ibid.*: p. 150.

13. Starzl, T. E., Waddell, W. R., and Marchioro, T. L.: Quoted *in* Med Trib, Apr 25–26, 1964, p. 9.

14. Freund, P. A.: Ethical problems in human experimentation, New Eng J Med 273:687, 691 (Sep 23), 1965.

15. *Ibid.*

16. Med Trib: Sep 18–19, 1965, pp. 24–25.

17. *Ibid.*: Nov 28–29, 1964, p. 7.

18. *Ibid.*: Sep 11–12, 1965, p. 8.

19. Freund, P. A.: See ref. 14, *supra*, p. 692.

20. *Ibid.*: p. 689.

21. *Kaiser* vs *Suburban Transportation System*, 398 P.2d 14, 1965.

CHAPTER 11

1. Woolf, Virginia: See ref. 5, chap. 2; Woolf, Leonard: Beginning Again, New York, Harcourt, 1964, p. 82.

2. AMA News: Jan 9, 1961, p. 10.

3. Report: p. 183.

4. *Ibid.*

5. Challener, W. A.: The law of sexual sterilization in Pennsylvania, 57 Dick. L. Rev. 298, 1952, cited in Report, p. 184.

6. Report: pp. 187–188, concerning *Buck* vs *Bell*, 274 U.S. 200, 1927.

7. *Ibid.*: p. 187.

8. New Med Mat: Nov 1962, pp. 17, 22.

9. Birnbaum, M.: Eugenic sterilization, JAMA *175*:951, 1961.

10. Bass, M. S.: Marriage for the mentally deficient, Ment Retard 2:198 (Aug), 1964. See also the same author's Marriage, parenthood, and prevention of pregnancy, Amer J Ment Defic *68*:318, 1963, and Sex education for the handicapped, Family Life Coordinator *13*:59, 1964.

11. Ref. 2, *supra*: MWN, Mar 30, 1962, p. 25; New Med Mat, Aug, 1962, p. 35.

12. Ref. 2, *supra*.

13. Johnson, M. H.: Social and psychological effects of vasectomy, Amer J Psychiat *121*:482, 1964.

14. *Ball* vs *Mudge*, 391 P.2d 201, 1964; for a similar statement in a Pennsylvania case, see *Shaheen* vs *Knight*, 6 Lycoming 19, 11 Penn. D & C 2d 41, 1957, where the court stated that "to allow damages for the normal birth of a normal child is foreign to the universal public sentiment of the people." Also article on Sterilization, consent and public policy, AMA News, Jan 23, 1961.

15. Birnbaum: See ref. 9, *supra*.

16. AMA Committee on Human Reproduction: The control of fertility, JAMA *194*:462, 469, 1965.

17. Long: pp. 201 ff.

18. Moritz and Stetler: p. 121.

19. Rosen, H.: Abortion, Today's Health, Apr, 1965, pp. 24 ff.; also, Abortion: the increasing involvement of psychiatry, Frontiers of Clin Psychiat 2:1 (Dec 1), 1965.

20. *Ibid*.

21. Niswander, K. R., and Klein, M.: Law versus practice in therapeutic abortion, AMA scientific program reported in Mod Med *33*:11–12 (July 5), 1965. Also see Niswander's elaboration of these views in Medicine, morality, and law in abortion, Med Opinion & Rev *1*:(#3)35, 1965, emphasizing that abortion is "the protection society owes" women who are victims of unwanted pregnancy.

22. Gold, E. M.: Survey reported in Med Trib, Oct 19, 1964, p. 1.

23. Hall, R. G.: Study reported in Med Trib, May 1–2, 1965, p. 12.

24. Letter of Bronstein, S. B.: To AMA News, May 31, 1965, p. 4.

25. An Abortion Fact Sheet: Look, Oct 19, 1965, p. 150.

26. American Law Institute Model Penal Code: Tent. Draft No. 9, §207.11, Philadelphia, Amer Law Inst, May 8, 1959, p. 144.

27. Patricia Maginnis, quoted in Star, J.: The growing tragedy of illegal abortion, Look, Oct 19, 1965, pp. 149, 158.

28. Med Trib: Sep 20, 1965, p. 2; see also MWN, Oct 22, 1965, p. 70.

29. Long says that at common law the state was obliged to allege and prove that the woman was "quick with child" (the fetus had developed to the point where the mother was conscious of its movements) to establish the crime of abortion. The procuring of abortion before quickening was not a crime even though it constituted a grave moral wrong. In all United States jurisdictions, statutes dealing with abortion do not differentiate between abortions early or late in pregnancy; any expulsion of the fetus before it can sustain an independent existence is an abortion and a criminal act unless necessary to preserve the life of the mother (21 states), to save the life of the mother (seven states), or to preserve the life of the mother or child (nine states). (Since an abortion is the expulsion of the fetus, taking the baby before term as in a Caesarean section is, technically, an abortion, and this accounts for those statutes that

justify abortions necessary to preserve the life of the child.) Another eleven jurisdictions require either the need to save the life of the mother, or alternatively to proof of this, the certificates of one or two licensed physicians that such is the case.

Only seven jurisdictions have extraordinary abortion statutes. In Louisiana, any act to induce an abortion, without exception, is a crime even if an abortion does not result. In Massachusetts and Pennsylvania, a wilful or unlawful abortion is a crime and there is no specific exception—as in most statutes—concerning preserving the life of the mother (although the term "unlawful abortion" implies that under some circumstances abortions are lawful, and doctors in these states do perform therapeutic abortions). New Jersey provides that any abortion that is malicious or without justification is a crime. The District of Columbia has a liberal abortion law, providing that an abortion is within the exception if it is necessary to preserve the life or the health of the mother. Two jurisdictions, although less liberal than this, are more liberal than other jurisdictions; Colorado and New Mexico permit abortions if necessary to preserve the life of the mother or to prevent serious and permanent bodily injury to her. Although some statutes speak of preserving the life of the mother and others of saving her life, apparently there is no substantial difference between these two types of statute. For lists that cover all jurisdictions, see Stetler and Moritz, pp. 93–94.

30. Goldmark, C., Jr.: Inaugural address, Med Trib, Nov 8, 1965, p. 3.

31. Pflum, F. A.: Letter to JAMA *193*:1128, 1965.

32. Sonne, J. C.: Feticide as acting out, Voices *2*:1, Spring, 1966.

33. The Philadelphia Inquirer: Nov 29, 1965, p. 6; AMA News, Dec 13, 1965, p. 1.

34. The Wall Street Journal: Dec 2, 1965, p. 6.

CHAPTER 12

1. *Lynch* vs *Knight*, 9 H.L.C. 577, 598, 1861, 11 Eng. Rep. 854.

2. Prosser: p. 180.

3. *I de S et ux.* vs *W de S*, Y.B. 22 Edw. III, 1348, f. 99, pl. 60.

4. *Gillespie* vs *Brooklyn Heights R. Co.*, 178 N.Y. 347, 70 N.E. 857, 1904, 66 L.R.A. 618.

5. *Barbknecht* vs *Great Northern R. Co.*, 55 N.D. 104, 212 N.W. 776, 1927.

6. Prosser: p. 40.

7. *Dulieu* vs *White and Sons*, 2 K. B. 669, 1901, 70 L. J. (K. B. D.) 837.

8. *Hill* vs *Kimball*, 76 Tex. 210, 13 S.W. 59, 1890, 7 L.R.A. 618.

9. Goodrich, H. F.: Emotional disturbance as legal damage, 20 Mich. L. Rev. 497, 1922.

10. Y. B. 7 Edw. IV, f. 2, pl. 2.

11. *Basely* vs *Clarkson*, 3 Lev. 37, 1681.

12. *Mitchell* vs *Rochester R. Co.*, 45 N.E. 354, 1896, 34 L.R.A. 781, 56 Am. St. Rep. 604.

13. *Spade* vs *Lynn & Boston R. Co.*, 168 Mass. 285, 288, 47 N.E. 88, 89, 1897, 38 L.R.A. 512, 60 Am. St. Rep. 393.

14. Morris, C.: Morris on Torts, Brooklyn, Foundation Press, 1953, p. 199.

15. *Lynch* vs *Knight*, See ref. 1; *Falzone* vs *Busch*, 45 N.J. Sup. Ct. 559, 1965; *Caposella* vs *Kelley*, 154 N.Y.C.J. 17, 1965.

16. *Mitchell* vs *Rochester R. Co.*, See ref. 12.

17. Prosser: pp. 38–39.

18. *Ashby* vs *White*, 2 Ld. Raym. 938, 955, 1703.

19. Magruder, C.: Mental and emotional disturbance in the law of torts, 49 Harv. L. Rev. 1033, 1936.

20. Usdin, G. L.: Neurosis Following Trauma, *in* Bear, L. A., ed.: Law, Medicine, Science and Justice, Springfield (Ill.), Thomas, 1964, p. 236.

21. Kardiner, A.: Traumatic Neuroses of War, *in* American Handbook of Psychiatry, New York, Basic, 1959, p. 246.

22. Webster's Third New International Dictionary, unabridged, Springfield (Mass), Merriam, 1964.

23. Smith, H. W., and Solomon, H. C.: Traumatic neuroses in court, 30 Va. L. Rev. 87, 1943.

24. Thompson, G. N.: Post-traumatic psychoneurosis—a statistical survey, Amer J Psychiat *121*:1043 (May), 1965.

25. Brosin, H. W.: See ref. 21, p. 1177.

26. Harper, E. O.: Traumatic Neurosis, *in* Schroeder, O., Jr., ed.: The Mind: A Law-Medicine Problem, Cincinnati, Anderson, 1962, p. 333.

27. *Astle* vs *Olmstead*, 199 Okla. 498, 187 P. 2d 997, 1947.

28. *Davis* vs *Cleveland R. Co.*, 135 Ohio St. 401, 21 N.E. 2d 169, 1939.

29. Round Table Meeting: Neurosis and Trauma, Amer Psychiat Assn, Atlantic City, NJ, May 10, 1960.

30. Smith and Solomon: See ref. 23.

31. Thompson: See ref. 24.

32. *Mickelson* vs *Fischer*, 142 Pac. 1160, 1914.

33. Curran: p. 291.

34. Siegal: p. 65.

35. Usdin: See ref. 20, p. 234; also ref. 29.

36. Thompson: See ref. 24.

37. Round Table Meeting: See ref. 29.

38. Bohlen, F. H., and Polikoff, H.: Liability in Pennsylvania for physical effects of fright, 80 U. Pa. L. Rev. 627, 637, 1932.

39. Cheit, E. F.: Injury and Recovery in the Course of Employment, New York, Wiley, 1961, pp. 10–13.

40. Morris: See ref. 14, p. 340.

41. Simpson, R. A.: Costlier injuries, Wall Street Journal, July 27, 1965, p. 1.

42. *Lumberman's Casualty Co.* vs *Industrial Accident Commission*, 29 Cal 2d 492, 1946.

43. Case noted by Waters, T. C.: Mental illness: is it compensable?, Arch Environ Health (Chicago) 5:178, 1962.

44. Brill, N. Q., and Glass, J. F.: Workmen's compensation for psychiatric disorders, JAMA *193*:345, 1965.

45. *Carter* vs *General Motors*, 361 Mich 577, 106 N.W.2d 105, 1960.

46. *Trombley* vs *Michigan*, 366 Mich 649, 115 N.W.2d 561, 1962.

47. *Lehman* vs *Winterer Company*, 136 N.W.2d 649, 1965; *National Stores, Inc.* vs *Hunter*, CCH Workmen's Compensation Decisions, ¶4146, p. 3059 (Ky. Ct. of App. June 11, 1965); *Mannell* vs *Jerome*, CCH Workmen's Compensation Decisions, ¶2739, p. 691 (Kan. Supreme Ct., May 15, 1965).

CHAPTER 13

1. Prosser: p. 140.

2. *Ibid.*: pp. 48 ff.

3. *Ibid.*: pp. 34–37.

4. Report: p. 44.

5. *Ibid.*

6. *Ibid.*

7. Deutsch: pp. 418–419.

8. Report: p. 16.

9. NIMH: See ref. 11, chap. 5.

10. World Health Organization: Hospitalization of Ment Patients, 1955, p. 15.

11. Med Trib: Nov 7, 1960, p. 2.

12. Ref. 10: *supra.*

13. Commonwealth of Pennsylvania: Dept of Pub Welfare, Office of the Commissioner of Ment Health, Form MH 49–2–63 (25).

14. Report: p. 108.

15. Ref. 13: *supra.*

16. Myers, J. Martin, MD: Staff Letter, Med Director, Institute of the Pennsylvania Hosp, Apr 19, 1965.

17. Report: p. 111. The New York, Tennessee, and Wyoming laws are more recent.

18. Curran, W. J.: Progress in Mental Health Legislation, Speech delivered at 17th Ann'l Ment Hosp Institute, San Francisco, Sep 28, 1965; McGarry, A. L.: From coercion to consent, Law-Medicine Notes, N Eng J Med *274*:39, 1966.

19. Report: p. 114.

20. *Ibid.*: p. 38.

21. *Ibid.*: pp. 94–99.

22. *Ibid.*: p. 39.

23. Ref. 21: *supra*; also see District of Columbia Hospitalization of the Ment Ill Act, Sep 15, 1964, §21–355 (c).

24. Lebensohn, Z. M., MD: Editorial, Med Ann DC *29*:505, 1960.

25. Science Fortnightly: Apr 29, 1964, p. 3.

26. Report: p. 31.

27. *Ibid.*: pp. 32–35, 68–70, where nine states are listed. Illinois and New York in 1964 and 1965 began use of medical commitment procedures, Illinois Ment Health Code of 1963, effective July 1, 1964; New York Ment Hygiene Law of 1964, effective Sep 1, 1965.

28. *State* vs *Mullinax*, 269 S.W.2d 72, 1954.

29. Pennsylvania Ment Health Act of 1951: P.L. 533, as amended Article I, Section 102 (13); Article III, Sections 311 and 312.

30. Report: p. 35.

31. *Ibid.*: p. 37.

32. New York Ment Hygiene Law of 1964, effective Sep 1, 1965.

33. Ref 18: *supra.*

34. District of Columbia Hospitalization of the Mentally Ill Act: Sep 15, 1964.

35. Ref 18: *supra.*

36. Follow-up Study of 378 Patients: Conducted by Wilder, J. F., Zwerling, I., and Levin, G., reported in Psychiat Progress, Nov, 1965.

37. Leifer, R.: Assistant Professor of Psychiat, State Univ of NY, Upstate Med Center, Syracuse, speech to Amer Psychological Assn, reported in Med Trib, Oct. 4, 1965, p. 1; see also Dr. Leifer's letter to the editor, Med Trib, Oct 23–24, 1965, p. 4.

CHAPTER 14

1. Peal, J.: Meeting, Golden Gate Group Psychotherapy Soc, San Francisco, June 13, 1964, reported in Psychiat Spectator *1*:(≢12)11(Sep), 1964.

2. Council of State Governments: The Mental Health Programs of the Forty-eight States, 1950, p. 69.

3. Report: p. 142.

4. Pennsylvania Mental Health Act of 1951: P.L. 533, as amended.

5. Lebensohn, Z. M.: American psychiatry and the general hospital, Med Ann DC *33*:47, 1964.

6. Pokorny, A.: General hospital psychiatry, Ment Hosp *14*:87, 1964.

7. Report: pp. 158–162.

8. *Ibid.*: p. 143.

9. Royal Commission on the Law Relating to Mental Illness and Mental Deficiency, 1954–57: Report, CMD. No. 169, §299, p. 103, 1957.

10. NIMH: See ref. 11, chap. 5.

11. Report: pp. 158–162.

12. Ref. 4: *supra*, Article VIII, §801 (5).

13. Report: pp. 158–162.

14. *Ibid.*: These states are Idaho, Missouri, New Mexico, North Dakota, Ohio, Oklahoma, South Carolina, Texas and Utah.

15. Louisiana, North Dakota and Pennsylvania are the other states specifically allowing visitation rights to ministers.

16. Connecticut, Louisiana, Massachusetts, North Dakota, Pennsylvania, Rhode Island and Vermont.

17. Report: p. 161, fn. 7.

18. Ref. 4: *supra*, Article VIII, §801 (7).

19. Report: p. 162, fn. 27.

20. Ref. 4: *supra*, Article VIII, §801 (1).

21. Ref. 16: *supra*.

22. Colorado, Illinois, Kentucky, New York, Texas and Wisconsin. In addition, Louisiana and Pennsylvania, already listed as states having statutory provision regarding right of patient to be visited by counsel, also have statutory provisions regarding right to write to counsel; they are the only states providing both of these rights.

23. Deutsch: pp. 216–217.

24. Lebensohn, Z. M.: Impressions of hospital psychiatry in Holland, Ment Hosp *7*:(no. 8)22,26, 1956, *in* Report, p. 146.

25. Report: p. 147.

26. *Ibid.*: pp. 163–164.

27. Birnbaum, M.: Eugenic sterilization, JAMA *175*:951, 957, 1961.

28. ———: Speech reported in Med Trib, Aug 5, 1964, p. 31.

29. Report: p. 128.

30. Pinel, P.: Treatise on Insanity, Davis, D. D., trans., New York, Hafner, 1962, pp. 216–217.

31. MWN: Oct 15, 1965, p. 135.

32. Hundziak, M., and Pasamanick, B.: Occupational and industrial therapy in the treatment of psychiatric patients: a controlled study of efficacy in an intensive treatment institution, Genetic Psychology Monographs 69, Provincetown (Mass), Journal Press, 1964, pp. 41–42.

33. Report: p. 151.

34. Goldman, R. P., and Ross, S.: The patients who shouldn't be in, Parade (part 1), Nov 11, 1956, p. 17.

35. Cleary, D. M.: The Philadelphia Evening Bulletin, June 16, 1965, pp. 1, 68; Med Trib, Aug 16, 1965, p. 23.

36. Report: p. 151.

37. Bartlett, F. L.: Institutional peonage: our exploitation of mental patients, Atlantic Monthly, July, 1964, p. 116.

38. Report: p. 151.

39. *Ibid.*: pp. 150–151, table p. 166. The nine states requiring postadmission examinations are Idaho, Missouri, New Mexico, New York, North Dakota, South Carolina, Tennessee, Utah and Virginia; the twelve requiring periodic examinations thereafter are Arizona, Louisiana, Maine, Missouri, New Mexico, New York, North Dakota, South Carolina, Tennessee, Texas, Utah, and West Virginia. The District of Columbia Act of Sep 15, 1964, also provides for periodic examinations.

40. *Muhlmichl* vs *State of New York*, 247 N.Y.S. 2d 959, 1964.

41. *Williams* vs *State*, 260 N.Y.S.2d 953, 1965.

42. Factor: Feb 2, 1962, p. 1.

CHAPTER 15

1. Bazelon, D. L.: Speech to Conf on State Mental Health Planning, reported *in* Lederer, E.: Crime needs psychiatry, Sci News Letter *87*:147 (Mar 6), 1965.

2. Cormier, B.: Speech to Third World Congress of Psychiatry, Med News, June 30, 1961, p. 23.

3. Davidson, H. A.: Speech to First Interamerican Conf on Legal Med and Forensic Science, Med Trib, Jan 18, 1963, pp. 1, 31.

4. Report: pp. 310–311.

5. *Ibid.*: p. 299.

6. *Ibid.*: p. 311.

7. Guttmacher and Weihofen: pp. 111–112; Curran: p. 639.

8. Report: p. 300 ff., table pp. 319–329.

9. Birnbaum, M.: Some questions that a lawyer may ask a psychiatrist concerning 'The Psychopath before the Law', New Eng J Med *261*:1223, 1959. The case is *In re Maddox*, 351 Mich Reports 358, 1958.

10. Report: p. 301, table pp. 319–329.

11. *Ibid.*

12. Gray, K. G., and Mohr, J. W.: Follow-up of Male Sexual Offenders, *in* Slovenko, Ralph, ed.: Sexual Behavior and the Law, Springfield (Ill.), Thomas, 1965, pp. 754–755.

13. Slovenko, R.: *ibid.*, note p. 757.

14. Macdonald, J. M.: Psychiatry and the Criminal, Springfield (Ill.), Thomas, 1958, p. 124.

15. Slovenko, R.: Quoting Bowman, Karl M., and Engle, Bernice, ref. 12, *supra*, p. 115.

16. Macdonald: Ref. 14 *supra*, p. 124.

17. Report: p. 310.

18. Governor's Study Commission on the Deviated Criminal Sex Offender, Michigan, 1951, p. 168.

19. Gordon, S.: Address to panel at Federal Bar Assn Convention, *in* Gordon, H. Y.: Law parley told of failure in treating delinquents, The Philadelphia Evening Bulletin, Sep 24, 1963, p. 100.

20. Golden, J. S., Silver, R. J., and Marchionne, A. M.: Process juvenile delinquents: description of a dissolute type, presented at Divisional Meeting, Amer Psychiat Assn, Philadelphia, Nov 20–21, 1964, reported in Psychiat Spectator *2*:6 (Apr), 1965.

21. Time: Aug 21, 1964, p. 65.

22. Forer, L. G.: Is juvenile court unjust to children? The Philadelphia Sunday Bulletin Magazine, June 20, 1965, p. 4.

23. Piliavin, I., and Briar, S.: Police encounters with juveniles, Amer J Sociol *70*:206, 1964.

24. Personal Glimpses: Reader's Digest, Sep, 1965, pp. 29–30.

CHAPTER 16

1. Savitt, R. A.: Psychoanalytic studies on addiction: ego structure in narcotic addiction, Psychoanal Quart *32*:(#1)56, 1963.

2. *Johnson* vs *Primm*, 396 P.2d 426, 1964.

3. Brooten, G.: *in* The Philadelphia Inquirer, Oct 29, 1965, p. 30.

4. Walsh, J.: *in* Science *149*:951–952 (Aug 27), 1965. In addition to the amphetamines and barbiturates covered by the law, the Food and Drug Administration, in January, 1966, proposed to control 17 other drugs; interested parties were given 30 days to submit their comments. The drugs were: *1.* those having a potential for abuse because of their depressant effect on the central nervous system: glutethimide (Doriden), chlordiazepoxide (Librium), perobamate (Miltown, Equanil, etc.), ethchlorvynol (Placidyl), choral hydrate, diazepam (Valium), ethinamate (Valmid), methyprylon (Noludar), paraldehyde; *2.* those having a potential for abuse and habit-formation because of their stimulant effect on the central nervous system: "D" and "DL" methamphetamine and their salts, phenmetrazine (Preludin); and *3.* those having a potential for abuse because of their hallucinatory effect (which drugs are not legally available in drug stores): D-lysergic acid diethylamide (LSD-25), peyote, mescaline and its salts, dimethyltryptamine (DMT), psilocyn, psilocybin. AMA News, Jan 24, 1966, p. 6.

5. ———: See ref. 4, *supra.*

6. Science *145*:1418 (Sep 27), 1964.

7. Hamburger, E.: Barbiturate use in narcotic addicts, JAMA *189*:366, 1964.

8. Smith, G. M., and Beecher, H. K.: Report to Amer Soc for Pharmacology and Experimental Therapeutics, MWN, Sep 25, 1964, p. 52.

9. Statement by AMA Council on Drugs and Committee on the Med Aspects of Sports: *in* JAMA *190*:adv p. 49, 1964.

10. Breitner, C.: Appetite suppressing drugs as an etiologic factor in mental illness, Psychosomatics *4*:327, 1963.

11. AMA News: Aug 3, 1964, p. 8.

12. Speech: Before the Amer Pub Health Assn, Med Trib, Oct 28, 1964.

13. The Jellinek formula is found in World Health Organization, Expert Committee on Mental Health (Alcoholism Sub-Committee), First Report, WHO Technical Report Series, No. 42, 1951, and Second Report, No. 48, 1952; see also Popham, R. E., and Schmidt, W.: Statistics of Alcohol Use and Alcohol in Canada, 1871–1956, Toronto, Univ of Toronto Press, 1958, Jones H.: Alcoholic Addiction: A Psycho-social Approach to Abnormal Drinking, London, Tavistock, 1963, pp. 5–7.

14. Keller, M.: Alcoholism: nature and extent of the problem, The Annals of the Amer Acad of Political and Social Sci *315*:2, 1958.

15. Mowrer, H. R.: A psychocultural analysis of the alcoholic, *in* McCarthy, R. G., ed.: Drinking and Intoxication, New Haven, Yale Center of Alcohol Studies, 1959, p. 297.

16. Jones: See ref. 13, *supra*, p. 15.

17. Williams, R. J.: Free and Unequal, Austin, Univ of Texas Press, 1953, pp. 103–106.

18. Jones: See ref 13, *supra*, p. 18.

19. Pattison, E. M.: Alcoholism, Psychiat Opinion, Summer, 1965, p. 39. See also Gerard, D. L., Saenger, G., and Wile, R.: The abstinent alcoholic, Arch Gen Psychiat *6*:99, 1962; Target, Dept of Health, Harrisburg, Pa, July, 1963, and Aug, 1965.

20. Burnett, W. H.: Legal processing of the alcoholic, paper presented at Nat'l Conf on Legal Issues in Alcoholism and Alcohol Usage, sponsored by Boston Univ Law-Medicine Institute, reported by Chayet, N. L.: N Eng J Med *273*:547, 1965.

21. *Ibid.*: p. 548.

22. Prosser: p. 127.

23. *Beverly's Case*, 76 Eng. Rep. 1118, K.B. 1603; see Report, p. 8.

24. Davidson: p. 163; also see 22 *CJS*, Criminal Law §§65–72, Brooklyn, Amer Law Book, 1961, pp. 213–223.

25. Time: Sep 24, 1965, p. 49.

26. Report: pp. 112–113.

27. *Ibid.*: pp. 107–108.

28. *Ibid.*: p. 21. Other estimates place this figure at 2% (see the same source, p. 19) or 3%. The latter figure is based on a 1962 census by the Pub Health Serv, US Dept of HEW; of 538,000 patients resident in mental institutions at the time, 16,300 carried the diagnosis of alcoholic. The difference between the utilization of private and public hospitals for treatment of alcoholics is demonstrated by figures of 1,700 of 13,000 patients in private institutions (or 14%) carrying the alcoholic designation, compared to 14,600 of 525,000 patients in public institutions (less than 3%).

29. New York Ment Hygiene Law: §307. Added L. 1965, C. 813, §1.

30. Pennsylvania Ment Health Act of 1951: P.L. 533, as amended, Article I, Section 102 (7).

31. *Ibid.*: Article III; Section 301 (3); Section 326 (a) (6), (b) (4); Section 329.

32. Letter to House Commerce Committee by Blasingame, F. J. L.: AMA Executive Vice President, AMA News, Oct 18, 1965, p. 6.

33. Waller, J. A.: Speech before Nat'l Conf on Legal Issues in Alcoholism and Alcohol Usage, AMA News, Aug 9, 1965, p. 8.

34. Drinking and driving: JAMA *167*:1499, 1958.

35. Selzer, M. L., and Weiss, S.: Alcoholism and fatal automobile accidents: study in futility, Psychiat Spectator *2*:(#7)1, 1965; Amer J Psychiat *122*:762, 1966.

36. Christie, N.: *in* Chayet, ref. 20, *supra*, p. 548.

37. Stetler and Moritz: pp. 288–289; AMA News, Oct 11, 1965, p. 13.

38. About a third of the states have specific blood-alcohol figures written into their codes. In a representative formulation a figure of between 0.05% and 0.15% (50 and 150 mg per 100 ml) is taken to mean that the driver is "possibly under the influence," final decision being based on clinical findings. A figure in excess of 0.15%, then, removes from the trial court the burden of deciding, on the basis of oral testimony, whether the driver was "under the influence." Davidson, p. 168. The proposed legislation in England and Canada, and that

proposed by Dr. Abraham Mirkin, Chairman of the AMA Committee on the Med Aspects of Automotive Safety, makes the alcohol blood level itself an offense rather than merely a test of the degree of intoxication of the driver. Lister, J.: By the London post, N Eng J Med *273*:758–759, 1965; AMA News, Oct 25, 1965, p. 3.

39. Selzer, M. L.: Alcoholism and traffic deaths, editorial in Med Trib, Sep 8, 1965, p. 15; AMA News, Oct 25, 1965, p. 3.

40. AMA News: Aug 23, 1965, p. 9.

41. Law-Medicine Notes: Narcotics, Treatment and Crime, from the Law-Medicine Institute, Boston Univ, N Eng J Med *271*:309, 1964.

42. Lindesmith, A. R.: The Addict and The Law, Bloomington, Indiana Univ. Press, 1965, p. 11.

43. *Ibid.*: p. 10.

44. *Ibid.*: pp. 223, 227.

45. Lewis, D. C., and Zinberg, N. E.: Narcotic usage: a historical prespective on a difficult medical problem, N Eng J Med *270*:1045, 1964.

46. Nyswander, M.: Drug Addiction, *in* American Handbook of Psychiatry, New York, Basic, 1959, p. 615.

47. The Harrison Act: 38 Stat. 785 (1914) as amended, 26 U.S.C. §4701.

48. Lindesmith: See ref. 42, *supra*, p. 31.

49. *Webb* vs *United States*, 249 U.S. 96, 1919.

50. *United States* vs *Behrman*, 258 U.S. 280, 1922.

51. *Linder* vs *United States*, 268 U.S. 5, 1925.

52. State of New Jersey, Executive Dept, Assembly Bill No. 488: Veto Message of Gov. Robert J. Meyner, mimeographed, June 28, 1956.

53. Lindesmith: See ref. 42, *supra*, chap. 4, for an analysis of the Federal Bureau of Narcotics statistics.

54. Vogel, V. H., Isbell, H., and Chapman, K. W.: Present status of narcotic addiction, JAMA *138*:1019, 1948.

55. Lindesmith: See ref. 42, *supra*, p. 122.

56. *Ibid.*

57. Med Trib: Oct 6, 1965, p. 23; The Washington Post, Nov 25, 1965, p. 83.

58. Javits, J. J.: Article on narcotics addiction, Med Trib, July 19, 1965, pp. 1, 16.

59. Dole, V. P., and Nyswander, M.: A medical treatment for diacetylmorphine (heroin) addiction, JAMA *193*:646, 1965.

60. Vogel, V. H.: Letter to the editor, The treatment of drug addiction, JAMA *194*:680, 1965.

61. The Synanon Foundation Story: Med Trib, Oct 12, 1965, p. 1, and Oct 14, 1965, p. 1. Also Alverson, C. E.: Kicking the habit, Wall Street Journal, Nov 10, 1965, p. 1.

62. Casselman, B. W.: *in* Drug addiction: five views on a vexing problem, Med Trib, Oct 9–10, 1965, pp. 8, 26.

63. *Robinson* vs *California*, 370 U.S. 660, 1962. See The cruel and unusual punishment clause and the substantive criminal law, Note: 79 Harv L Rev 635, 1966, which suggests that "*Robinson* raises more questions than it answers" and complains of "the Court's failure to provide a reasoned basis for its decision," although the case "does help point up the fact that the criminal law is basically intended to apply to—and that our notions of blameworthiness and deterrence turn on—the commission of voluntary acts," p. 655.

64. Law-Medicine Notes: See ref. 41, *supra*.

65. Editorial: Psychedelic drugs, Acad Reporter *10*:4 (Oct), 1965.

66. McCluskie, J. A. W., and Horne, C. H.: The food of the gods, Scot Med J *8*:489, 1963.

67. Ludwig, A. M., and Levine, J.: Patterns of hallucinogenic drug abuse, JAMA *191*:92, 1965.

68. Brodie, B. B., Prockop, D. J., and Shore, P. A.: An interpretation of the action of psychotropic drugs, Postgrad Med *24*:296, 1958.

69. Jarvik, M. E.: Psychopharmacology, *in* Kline, N. S., ed.: Amer Assn for the Advancement of Sci, No. 42, Washington, DC, 1956, p. 145.

70. Klerman, G. L.: Research programs which utilize psychotomimetic drugs: a psychiatrist's viewpoint, Psychiat Opinion, Fall, 1964, pp. 14–15.

71. Ludwig and Levine: See ref. 67, *supra.*

72. Baker, E. F. W.: The use of lysergic acid diethylamide (LSD) in psychotherapy, Canad Med Assn J *91*:1200, 1964.

73. Levine, J., and Ludwig, A. M.: Address to second Conf on the Use of LSD in Psychotherapy, Frontiers of Hospital Psychiatry *2*:3 (Aug 1), 1965.

74. Klerman: See ref. 70, *supra*, pp. 15–16.

75. Weil, A. T.: The strange case of the Harvard drug scandal, Look, Nov 5, 1963, p. 38.

76. Grinker, Sr., R. R.: Bootlegged ecstasy, editorial, JAMA *187*:768, 1964; Klerman, ref. 70, *supra*, p. 13.

77. Smith, H.: Do drugs have religious import? The Journal of Philosophy *61*:517, 1964.

78. Dahlberg, C. C.: Letter to the editor, Med Trib, Dec 30, 1964, p. 11.

79. New York Ment Hygiene Law: §429, Added L. 1965, c. 332, §4.

80. Plotnikoff, N., and Glasky, A. J.: Drug enhancement of nucleic acid synthesis, learning, and memory; paper read at Interdisciplinary Symposium in the Biological-Behavioral Sciences, 132nd AAAS Meeting, Berkeley, Cal, Dec 27, 1965; Science *150*:924, 1965; JAMA *195*:adv p. 31 (Jan 3), 1966.

CHAPTER 17

1. Med Trib: Sep 6, 1965, p. 23.

2. Editorial: New Eng J Med *273*:612, 1965.

3. *Hammonds* vs *Aetna Casualty & Surety Company*, 237 F. Supp 96, 1965, p. 101.

4. Davidson, H. A.: Speech, Arthur P. Noyes Memorial Conf, Norristown, Pa., Sep 18, 1965.

5. Rosen, E.: They shouldn't do this to doctors!, Med Economics, Sep 6, 1965, p. 213.

6. Sheridan, J.: Liability of Non-treating Physicians, Medicolegal Monograph, Law Department, AMA.

7. *Ibid.*

8. Goodman, A. J.: Letter to the editor, The New Republic, Jan 2, 1965, p.22.

9. Ref. 4, *supra.*

10. Opinion of Judicial Council, AMA: "General Walker and Dr. Smith," JAMA *185*:36, 1963.

11. Walker has won a $500,000 libel judgment in Fort Worth, Texas, against the Associated Press and a $3,000,000 libel judgment against the Associated Press and New Orleans Times-Picayune Publishing Corporation in Shreveport, Louisiana, on the ground that the AP report falsely described him as assuming command of Ole' Miss rioters and leading them in a charge against United States marshals. The AP has announced that it is appealing these awards.

12. AMA News: Oct 12, 1964, p. 1.
13. *Jenkins* vs *United States*, 307 F.2d 637, 1962.
14. Ridgeway, J.: The snoops: private lives and public service, The New Republic, Dec 19, 1964, p. 13.
15. Time: June 18, 1965.
16. Messaros, H.: The Philadelphia Sunday Bulletin, Feb 7, 1965, p. 25.
17. Grimes, J.: The Wall Street Journal, Apr 8, 1965, p. 1.
18. Outlook: MWN, June 11, 1965, p. 21.
19. Ridgeway, J.: Ref. 14, *supra*.
20. Sci News Letter: Sep 18, 1965, p. 183.
21. The New Republic: June 19, 1965, p. 8.
22. Cohen, L.: Clinical Psychology: Current Status, *in* Regan, P. F., ed.: Behavorial Science Contributions to Psychiatry, International Psychiatry Clinics, Boston, Little, April, 1965, p. 489.
23. Sci News Letter: See ref. 20, *supra*.
24. Flannery, T. A.: Speech at Northwestern Univ School of Law seminar, *in* Med Trib, Sep 4, 1961, p. 30.
25. Menninger, W. W., and English, J. T.: Confidentiality and the request for psychiatric information for nontherapeutic purposes, Amer J Psychiat *122*: 638, 1965.
26. *Ibid.*: p. 644.
27. Hartog, J.: Letter to the editor, The New Republic, Apr 10, 1965, p. 27.

CHAPTER 18

1. Benet, William Rose (ed.): See ref. 5, chap. 1, p. 506.
2. Principles of Medical Ethics, Opinions and Reports of the Judicial Council: JAMA (spec ed.), June 7, 1958, section 9.
3. Guttmacher and Weihofen: p. 276.
4. Stetler and Moritz: p. 270.
5. DeWitt, C.: Privileged Communications Between Physician and Patient, Springfield (Ill.), Thomas, 1958, p. 3.
6. *Ibid.*: pp. 4–5.
7. *Ibid.*: p. 7.
8. Tiemann, W. H.: The Right to Silence: Privileged Communication and the Pastor, Richmond, Knox, 1964, p. 92; DeWitt, see ref. 5, pp. 8–9.
9. *Alford* vs *Johnson*, 146 S.W. 516, 1912.
10. *Johnson* vs *Commonwealth*, 221 S.W.2d 87, 1949.
11. *Mullen* vs *United States*, 263 F.2d 275, 1959. This and the cases mentioned in refs. 9 and 10 are cited Tiemann, pp. 96–99.
12. Tiemann: See ref. 8, p. 116.
13. DeWitt: See ref. 5, p. 9.
14. *Ibid.*: See ref. 1.
15. *Duchess of Kingston's Case*, 20 How. St. Trials 355, 1776.
16. *Garner* vs *Garner*, 36 T.L.R. 196, 1920; see DeWitt, ref. 5, *supra*, pp. 12–13.
17. Zenoff, E.: Confidential and privileged communication, JAMA *182*:656–657, 1962.
18. Friedman, G. A.: Medical confidences and the law, Resident Physician 4:132–133, 1958.
19. See ref. 38, *infra*.
20. *Berry* vs *Moench*, 331 P. 2d 814, 1959.

21. *Simonsen* vs *Swenson*, 177 N.W. 831, 1920, 9 A.L.R. 1250.

22. GAP Report: p. 92.

23. Freud, S.: The Interpretation of Dreams, 1890 (1900), (standard ed.), vol. 4, London, Hogarth, 1958, pp. 100–101. Freud's view of the therapeutic effect of tracing the pathological idea back to the elements from which it originated represents an early phase in his theory of analytic therapy; later works do not regard uncovering of itself as necessarily therapeutic. For a discussion of this change in Freudian theory, see Arlow, J. A., and Brenner, C.: Psychoanalytic concepts and the structural theory, J Amer Psychoanal Assn Monograph Series No. 3, New York, Internat Univ Press, 1964. The instruction of the patient to shut his eyes was eliminated in later accounts by Freud of his technic.

24. Waelder, R.: Basic Theory of Psychoanalysis, New York, Internat Univ Press, 1960, pp. 237–238.

25. *Ibid.*: pp. 238–239.

26. Breuer, J., and Freud, S.: Studies on Hysteria, 1895, (standard ed.), vol. 2, London, Hogarth, 1955, p. 29.

27. "The case upon which I propose to report in the following pages (once again only in a fragmentary manner). . . .": Introductory Remarks, From the History of an Infantile Neurosis, 1918, (standard ed.), vol. 17, London, Hogarth, 1955, p. 7.

28. GAP Report: pp. 100, 106–107.

29. *Ibid.*: pp. 107–108.

30. *Ibid.*: pp. 106–107.

31. Adland, M. L.: Letter to editor, The Washington Post, Sep 24, 1960, p. A10.

32. MWN: Sep 1, 1961, p. 30.

33. The Washington Post: Dec 22, 1960, p. C1.

34. Lebensohn, Z. M.: Editorial, Psychiatry and national security, JAMA *175*:1001, 1961.

35. Sidel, V.: Confidential information and the physician, New Eng J Med *264*:1133, 1961.

36. AMA News: Oct 11, 1965, p. 12.

37. GAP Report: pp. 111–112.

38. *Binder* vs *Ruvell*, Civil Docket 52C2535, Circuit Court of Cook County, Ill., June 24, 1952; see ref. 3, p. 269; see Comment 47 N.W.U.L. Rev. 384, 1952.

39. Zenoff: See ref. 17, p. 660.

40. GAP Report: p. 98.

41. *Clark* vs *Geraci*, 208 N.Y.S.2d 654, 1960; Med News, Mar 10, 1961, p. 12.

42. Chávez, I.: Professional ethics in medicine in our time, JAMA *190*:226, 1964.

43. GAP Report: p. 105.

44. Zenoff: See ref. 17, p. 659. "Within the last decade, nine states have adopted laws granting privilege to the communications between psychologists and their clients. It is noteworthy that two of these states, New Hampshire and Tennessee, have no physician-patient privilege laws. Until 1959, when Georgia adopted a psychiatrist-patient privilege—and, incidentally, became the first state to do so—it, also, was one of the states which had a psychologist-client but not a physician-patient privilege."

45. O'Neill, M. J.: Capital rounds, MWN, Sep 24, 1965, p. 90.

Indexes

Index of Cases

The numbers in parentheses refer to bibliographic references.

Index of Names

Index of Subjects